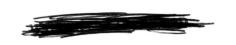

GLAUCOMA NEUROPROTECTION

GLAUCOMA NEUROPROTECTION

ROBERT N. WEINREB, MD

Distinguished Professor of Ophthalmology
Director, Hamilton Glaucoma Center
University of California, San Diego
La Jolla, California

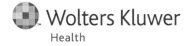
Wolters Kluwer

Health

Project Manager: Jennifer Jett
Executive Director of Continuing Education: James T. Magrann
Production Services: Maryland Composition Co., Inc.
Printer: Kugler Publications

Printed in the Netherlands

Library of Congress Cataloging-in-Publication Data

Weinreb, Robert N., 1949-
  Glaucoma neuroprotection / Robert N. Weinreb.
    p. ; cm.
  Includes bibliographical references.
  ISBN 0-7817-6350-9
  1. Glaucoma—Treatment.   2. Optic nerve—Diseases—Treatment.   3. Neuroophthalmology.
I. Title.
  [DNLM: 1. Glaucoma—prevention & control. 2. Neurodegenerative Diseases—prevention & control. WW 290 W423g 2006]
  RE871.W34 2006
  617.7'41—dc22

                                                                    2005033111

    For questions regarding this continuing medical education activity, please contact the Wolters Kluwer Health Office of Continuing Education, 770 Township Line Road, Suite 300, Yardley, PA 19067; by phone: (215)521-8635; or by fax: (215)521-8637.
                                                        10 9 8 7 6 5 4 3 2 1

CONTENTS

GLAUCOMA NEUROPROTECTION
CME OVERVIEW

Release date
February 2006

Accreditation
Wolters Kluwer Health is accredited by the Accreditation Council for Continuing Medical Education to provide continuing medical education for physicians.

Credit Designation
Wolters Kluwer Health designates this educational activity for up to 5 category 1 credits toward the AMA Physician's Recognition Award. Each physician should claim only those credits that he/she actually spent in the activity. **AMA/PRA Category 1 credit is available only to U.S.-licensed physicians (MDs or DOs).**

Commercial Support
This CME activity is supported by an unrestricted educational grant from Allergan Pharmaceuticals, Inc.

Target Audience
This CME activity is intended for glaucoma specialists, clinical and academic ophthalmologists, and other physicians interested in the diagnosis and management of glaucoma.

Statement of Need
Glaucoma is the second leading cause of blindness worldwide.[1] In the U.S., more than 7 million office visits occur per year to monitor patients who have glaucoma or are at risk of developing the disease. Blindness from all forms of glaucoma in the U.S. is estimated to cost in excess of $1.5 billion annually. Furthermore, a substantial proportion of individuals remain either undiagnosed or inadequately treated, so the scope of the problem is probably even larger than the statistics suggest.[2] The number of individuals suspected of having glaucoma is believed to far exceed the number who have already been diagnosed. The magnitude of the problem is expected to increase in the coming years as the population ages.[1]

For more than a century, glaucoma treatment has been directed at lowering intraocular pressure (IOP). However, in the past few years, there have been significant advances in understanding the mechanisms for death of retinal neurons and in the development of neuroprotective therapies for glaucoma and other neurodegenerative diseases, such as Alzheimer's disease.

"Despite IOP-lowering treatment, patients with glaucoma often continue to progress," said Robert N. Weinreb, MD, Distinguished Professor and Director of the Hamilton Glaucoma Center at the University of California, San Diego. "Neuroprotection offers the possibility of further slowing the rate of progression and preventing blindness."[3] A full understanding of the mechanisms of neuroprotection, the preclinical animal models used to study glaucoma treatments, the findings of clinical trials, and the measures of glaucoma progression is necessary to evaluate potential neuroprotective treatments for patients with chronic open-angle glaucoma.

In July 2005, a symposium on neuroprotection in glaucoma was presented in Vienna, Austria at the World Glaucoma Congress, hosted by the AIGS. The audience, which consisted largely of general ophthalmologists who encounter glaucoma in the course of their practice, expressed a strong interest in learning more about the basic science and clinical relevance of neuroprotection research. Specifically, the participants asked about the relevance of experimental models for human primary open-angle glaucoma, the credibility of the experimental data to date, the levels of glutamate which cause cell damage, the cell types affected earliest in glaucoma, criteria to use when evaluating neuroprotective compounds, and the

incorporation of neuroprotection into a treatment pattern.

A summary of the Neuroprotection in Glaucoma symposium described above is being offered as a continuing medical education program in two formats—print and DVD—to accommodate individual differences in learning styles. Research on preferences for CME delivery modes has shown that next to in-person conferences, physicians prefer self-directed study programs in print-based and electronic formats.[4] In this program, the traditional printed book format provides detailed written summaries of each presentation, references, and a selection of the key visuals.

REFERENCES

1. Quigley HA, Vitale S. Models of open-angle glaucoma prevalence and incidence in the United States. *Invest Ophthalmol Vis Sci* 1997;38:83–91.
2. Weinreb RN, Khaw PT. Primary open-angle glaucoma. *Lancet* 2004; 363: 1711–1720.
3. Weinreb RN, Levin LA. Is neuroprotection a viable therapy for glaucoma? *Arch Ophthalmol* 1999;117:1540–1544.
4. Mamary E, Charles P. Promoting self-directed learning for continuing medical education. *Med Teach* 2003;25: 188–190.

Faculty Credentials and Disclosure Information

Editor
Robert N. Weinreb, MD
Distinguished Professor of Ophthalmology
Director, Hamilton Glaucoma Center
University of California, San Diego
La Jolla, California

Dr. Weinreb has disclosed that he had/has the following financial relationships/interests with commercial companies pertaining to this educational activity:
Consultant/Advisor: Allergan, Alcon, Pfizer, Merck, Zeiss-Meditec

Faculty
Joseph Caprioli, MD
Chief, Glaucoma Division
Jules Stein Eye Institute
University of California, Los Angeles
Los Angeles, California

Dr. Caprioli has disclosed that he had/has the following financial relationships/interests with commercial companies pertaining to this educational activity:
Grant/Research Funding: Alcon, Allergan
Consultant/Advisor: Allergan, Merck, Pfizer
Speakers Bureau: Merck, Allergan, Pfizer, Alcon

Prof. Lutz Frölich, MD, PhD
Professor of Geriatric Psychiatry
University of Heidelberg,
Mannheim, Germany

Prof. Frölich has disclosed that he had/has the following financial relationships/interests with commercial companies pertaining to this educational activity:
Grant/Research Funding: Lundbeck, Pfizer
Consultant/Advisor: AstraZeneca, Myriad, Nomad, Pfizer, Janssen-Cilag

David Garway-Heath, MD, FRCO phth
Consultant Ophthalmologist and Clinical Research Lead
Glaucoma Research Unit
Moorfields Eye Hospital
London, UK

Dr. Garway-Heath has disclosed that he had/has the following financial relationships/interests with commercial companies pertaining to this educational activity:
Consultant/Advisor: Carl Zeiss Meditec

Ivan Goldberg, MD
Glaucoma Service and Visiting Ophthalmologist
Sydney Eye Hospital
University of Sydney
Sydney, New South Wales, Australia

Dr. Goldberg has disclosed that he had/has the following financial relationships/interests with commercial companies pertaining to this educational activity:
Grant/Research Funding: Alcon, Allergan, Pfizer, Carl Zeiss Meditec, Glaukos
Consultant/Advisor: Alcon, Allergan, Pfizer
Speakers Bureau: Alcon, Allergan, Inc., Pfizer, Laserex

David Greenfield, MD
Associate Professor of Ophthalmology
University of Miami School of Medicine
Bascom Palmer Eye Institute
Miami, Florida

Dr. Greenfield has disclosed that he had/has the following financial relationships/interests with commercial companies pertaining to this educational activity:
Grant/Research Funding: Carl Zeiss Meditec, Heidelberg Engineering, Allergan
Consultant/Advisor: Alcon, Allergan, Pfizer
Speakers Bureau: Alcon, Allergan, Pfizer

William A. Hare, OD, PhD
Research Investigator, Program Team
  Leader
Department of Biological Sciences
Allergan, Inc.
Irvine, California

Dr. Hare has disclosed that he had/has the following financial relationships/interests with commercial companies pertaining to this educational activity:
Stock Shareholder: Allergan
Other: Allergan employee

Theodore Krupin, MD
Clinical Professor of Ophthalmology
Feinberg School of Medicine
Northwestern University
Chicago, Illinois

Dr. Krupin has disclosed that he had/has the following financial relationships/interests with commercial companies pertaining to this educational activity:
Grant/Research Funding: Alcon, Allergan, Pfizer

Consultant/Advisor: Allergan, Pfizer
Speakers Bureau: Alcon, Allergan, Merck, Pfizer

Ronald K. Lai, PhD
Principal Scientist
Department of Biological Sciences
Allergan, Inc.
Irvine, California

Dr. Lai has disclosed that he had/has the following financial relationships/interests with commercial companies pertaining to this educational activity:
Other: Allergan employee

Leonard A. Levin, MD, PhD
Associate Professor of Ophthalmology
  and Visual Sciences, Neurology and
  Neurological Surgery
University of Wisconsin Medical School
Madison, Wisconsin

Dr. Levin has disclosed that he had/has the following financial relationships/interests with commercial companies pertaining to this educational activity:
Consultant/Advisor: Alcon, Allergan, Pfizer, Univalor, Merck, Inspire

Jeffrey M. Liebmann, MD
Clinical Professor of Ophthalmology
New York University School of Medicine
New York, New York

Dr. Liebmann has disclosed that he had/has the following financial relationships/interests with commercial companies pertaining to this educational activity:
Consultant/Advisor: Alcon, Allergan, Santen, Pfizer

Stuart Lipton, MD, PhD
Professor and Scientific Director
Neuroscience and Aging Center
Burnham Institute
La Jolla, California

Dr. Lipton has disclosed that he had/has the following financial relationships/interests with commercial companies pertaining to this educational activity:
Grant/Research Funding: Scios, Allergan, NeuroMolecular Pharmaceuticals
Consultant/Advisor: Scios, Allergan, Neuro-Molecular Pharmaceuticals, Chemicon, Forest Labs, Merck, Ortho Biotech (Johnson & Johnson)
Stock Shareholder: NeuroMolecular Pharmaceuticals (scientific founder)
Other: Advisor for MedaCorp and Gerson Lehrman Group Councils (financial consulting firms); Receives a share of royalties on Memantine patent

Manuel Vidal-Sanz, MD, PhD
Professor of Experimental Ophthalmology, Director of the Laboratory
of Experimental Ophthalmology and
Department Head
Department of Ophthalmology
Faculty of Medicine
University of Murcia
Murcia, Spain

Dr. Vidal-Sanz has disclosed that he had/has the following financial relationships/interests with commercial companies pertaining to this educational activity:
Grant/Research Funding: Allergan

Larry A. Wheeler, PhD
Senior Vice-President
Department of Biological Sciences
Allergan, Inc.
Irvine, California

Dr. Wheeler has disclosed that he had/has the following financial relationships/interests with commercial companies pertaining to this educational activity:
Other: Allergan employee

Elizabeth WoldeMussie, PhD
Research Investigator, Glaucoma Program
Department of Biological Sciences
Allergan, Inc.
Irvine, California

Dr. WoldeMussie has disclosed that she had/has the following financial relationships/interests with commercial companies pertaining to this educational activity:
Other: Allergan employee

Yeni H. Yücel, MD, PhD, FRCPC
(Neuropath)
Associate Professor
Department of Ophthalmology and Vision Sciences
Faculty of Medicine
University of Toronto
Toronto, Ontario, Canada

Dr. Yücel has disclosed that he had/has the following financial relationships/interests with commercial companies pertaining to this educational activity:
Grant/Research Funding: Allergan
Consultant/Advisor: Allergan

COI Peer Reviewers
Prof. Neville N. Osborne
Professor of Ocular Neurobiology
Department of Ophthalmology
Oxford, University
Oxford, UK

Prof. Osborne has disclosed that he has no financial relationship with or interests in any commercial company pertaining to this educational activity.

Stuart J. McKinnon, MD, PhD
Associate Professor of Ophthalmology
Department of Ophthalmology
Duke University Medical Center
Durham, North Carolina

Dr. McKinnon has disclosed that he had/has the following financial relationships/interests with commercial companies pertaining to this educational activity:
Consultant: Alcon
Speakers Bureau: Alcon, Pfizer

Medical Writing/Editorial Assistance
Mary C. Love
Medical Writer
Columbia, Maryland

Ms. Love has disclosed that she has no financial relationships with or interests in any commercial company pertaining to this educational activity.

Identification and Resolution of Faculty Conflict of Interests

Wolters Kluwer Health has identified and resolved any faculty conflicts of interest regarding this educational activity.

Off-label or Investigational Usage Discussion
The following faculty members have disclosed that their content discusses off-label usage of or unapproved drugs:

Dr. Lai: *Memantine has not been approved by the U.S. Food and Drug Administration for use in the treatment of glaucoma. Please consult product labeling for the approved usage of this drug or device.*

Dr. Lipton: *Memantine has not been approved by the U.S. Food and Drug Administration for use in the treatment of glaucoma. Please consult product labeling for the approved usage of this drug or device.*

Dr. Hare: *Memantine has not been approved by the U.S. Food and Drug Administration for use in the treatment of glaucoma. Please consult product labeling for the approved usage of this drug or device.*

Dr. Krupin: *Brimonidine has not been approved by the U.S. Food and Drug Administration for use in the treatment of glaucoma through neuroprotection. Please consult product labeling for the approved usage of this drug or device.*

Dr. Yücel: *Memantine has not been approved by the U.S. Food and Drug Administration for use in the treatment of glaucoma. Please consult product labeling for the approved usage of this drug or device.*

Dr. Wheeler: *Brimonidine has not been approved by the U.S. Food and Drug Administration for use in the treatment of glaucoma through neuroprotection. Please consult product labeling for the approved usage of this drug or device.*

Dr. WoldeMussie: *Memantine has not been approved by the U.S. Food and Drug Administration for use in the treatment of glaucoma. Please consult product labeling for the approved usage of this drug or device.*

Learning Objectives

After participating in this educational activity, physicians should be able to:

- Summarize the neurobiological rationale for neuroprotection.
- Describe the role of glutamate in neural degenerative diseases and the molecular mechanisms of neuroprotective agents that block glutamate excitotoxicity.
- Recall the methods for measuring neuroprotection and glaucoma progression in preclinical animal models and clinical trials.
- Explain the role of alpha-2 adrenergic system in neuronal survival.
- Recall the preclinical and clinical findings of drug therapies used for neuroprotection, including the alpha-2 agonists and the NMDA receptor antagonists.

Method of Physician Participation

To earn CME credit, a participant must read the monograph, comprehend the content, and complete the CME quiz and evaluation assessment survey on form printed at the end of the book, answering at least 70% of the CME quiz questions correctly. Participants must make a photocopy of the completed answer form for their own files and send their original answer form to Wolters Kluwer Health, Office of Continuing Education, 770 Township Line Road, Suite 300, Yardley, PA 19067. Only the first entry will be considered for credit and must be received by WKH by 2/28/2008. **Acknowledgment will be sent to participants within 6 to 8 weeks of participation. AMA/PRA Category 1 credit is available only to U.S.-licensed physicians (MDs or DOs). All other healthcare professionals who return the quiz and achieve a passing score will receive a certificate of completion for successful participation.**

Evaluation Method

Six evaluation assessment questions are included as part of the CME quiz. These questions ensure that WKH determines that each activity's learning objectives have been met, that the activity was of educational value to the target audience and was unbiased, assess whether or not the CME activity has resulted in a change in physician practice behavior, and offer participants a method of feedback.

Participation Expiration Date

February 28, 2008

NEUROBIOLOGIC RATIONALE FOR NEUROPROTECTION

LEONARD A. LEVIN, MD, PHD

There is a convincing rationale for the use of neuroprotection as a therapy for glaucoma from the neurobiologic point of view. This is based on the evidence that glaucoma is an optic neuropathy—specifically, a chronic axonal disease.

GLAUCOMA IS AN OPTIC NEUROPATHY

Glaucoma, as we now know, is not a disease of intraocular pressure (IOP). Traditionally, glaucoma was viewed as a disease of elevated IOP, in which visual loss could be prevented by lowering the pressure. Today, however, glaucoma is viewed as an optic nerve disease in which IOP is currently the most important risk factor available for change. Although lowering IOP has been linked with the prevention of visual loss in many patients, it has not been effective for all patients. Progression of disease despite a significant lowering of IOP has been demonstrated in all of the major, randomized clinical glaucoma trials, including the Advanced Glaucoma Intervention Study (AGIS),[1,2] the Collaborative Normal Tension Glaucoma Study,[3,4] the Collaborative Initial Glaucoma Treatment Study[5] Trial, and the Early Manifest Glaucoma Trial.[6]

Recent evidence indicates that variation in IOP over time is probably as important, if not more important, than the actual level of IOP for treated patients with glaucoma. A retrospective subanalysis of data from the AGIS showed that variation of pressure readings across office visits was more important than the absolute level of pressure.[7] Fluctuation in IOP over 24 hours could also be an independent risk factor for progression, but the evidence is less convincing[8,9] Asrani et al.[8] suggested that the diurnal IOP range and the IOP range over multiple days were significant risk factors for progression, even after adjusting for office IOP, age, race, gender, and visual field damage at baseline. In summary, glaucoma will progress even in patients with good pressure lowering.

Finally, lowering IOP could be good for the optic nerve in general—not only in glaucoma but also in other optic neuropathies. Thus, when glaucoma is treated by lowering the pressure, it may actually be treating the optic neuropathy, not just the elevated IOP.

On a neurobiologic basis, glaucoma fits into a classic pattern of a type of optic nerve diseases called "anterior optic neuropathies." This classification includes papilledema, anterior ischemic optic neuropathy, and disk drusen, as well as many more (Figs. 1-1 through 1-4). These anterior optic neuropathies have several common features, which are summarized in Table 1-1. The most important feature is the fact that the type of visual field defect is the nerve fiber bundle defect, unlike the defects in other optic neuropathies. They also share in common the death of retinal ganglion cells, the loss of the retinal nerve fiber layer, and optic atrophy.

The one feature of glaucoma that clearly separates it from these other diseases is that in glaucoma, the amount of cupping is much greater than the amount of pallor. The other diseases will typically show pallor to an extent greater than the amount of cupping. Other than that, glaucoma could be simply considered just

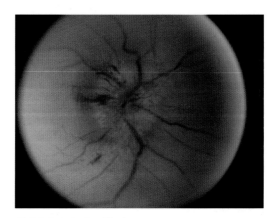

FIGURE 1-1. Papilledema.

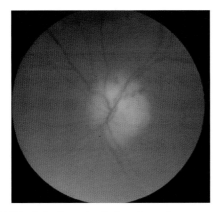

FIGURE 1-2. Anterior ischemic optic neuropathy.

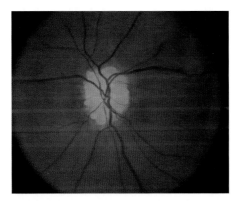

FIGURE 1-3. Disk drusen.

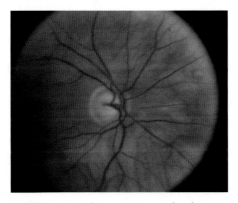

FIGURE 1-4. Primary open-angle glaucoma.

TABLE 1-1. COMMON FEATURES OF ANTERIOR OPTIC NEUROPATHIES

- Nerve fiber bundle visual field defects
- Death of retinal ganglion cells
- Loss of retinal nerve fiber
- Optic atrophy

one more anterior optic neuropathy, perhaps with a greater tendency to be associated with higher IOP in many cases.

There are several implications associated with thinking about glaucoma as an anterior optic neuropathy. First, neurons die in optic neuropathies—specifically the retinal ganglion cells, but also their direct and indirect targets in the brain. Also, neurons cannot divide and be replaced, except for rare cases in parts of the brain where there are stem cells. Most of the neurons in the central nervous system do not reproduce, and so the loss of the retinal ganglion cells cannot be replaced. Therefore, it is important to keep the neuron alive and functional, because the loss of function (i.e., the loss of vision) is irreversible. This process of keeping these cells alive and functional is called "neuroprotection" and constitutes a strategy for treating any of the optic neuropathies, including glaucoma.

GLAUCOMA IS A CHRONIC, AXONAL DISEASE

Glaucoma is not just an anterior optic neuropathy, but is also chronic and involves the axon.

In general, most optic neuropathies involve the axons and do not affect the cell bodies directly (Fig. 1-5).

A wealth of evidence exists that suggests glaucoma is primarily an axonal disease. The sites of the damage, changes in the lamina cribrosa, and disk hemorrhages all generally take place at the cup. In fact, the biomechanical evidence suggests that the major stresses are at the cup.[10]

Psychophysical evidence shows that as the visual field defects progress in glaucoma, the neural fiber bundle defects spread in a pattern representing changes at the disk (Fig. 1-6). If the spread were occurring at the ganglion cells, it would occur across the meridian

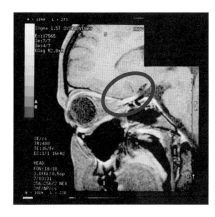

FIGURE 1-5. Optic neuritis. A patient with multiple sclerosis who developed inflammation of the optic nerve along the axons, as indicated by the white area contained within the red circle.

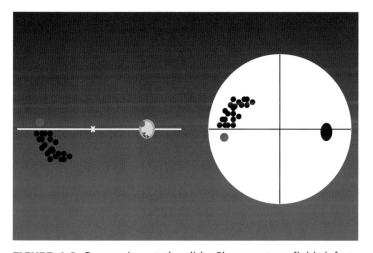

FIGURE 1-6. Progression at the disk. Glaucomatous field defects progress in patterns consistent with nerve fiber bundle injury and in most cases reflect injury occurring at the optic disk. Pattern of a superior nasal step field defect associated with damage at the inferotemporal disk and reflecting death of retinal ganglion cells in the inferotemporal retina (*black circles*). Crossover into the inferior nasal field (*red circle*) is unusual, because although the adjacent retinal ganglion cells in the superior retina are nearby, the corresponding superotemporal part of the disk is distant from the previously involved inferotemporal disk fibers (separated by the papillomacular bundle). In other words, the pattern of field progression is an indication that the locus of injury is primarily the disk.

in the adjacent ganglion cell, and would also occur across the visual field. However, that scenario is rarely seen. The progression takes place at the disk without crossing the horizontal meridian.[11,12]

Optic nerve diseases can be diseases of either the axon or the cell body. Anterior ischemic optic neuropathy and glaucoma are axonal, or white matter, diseases. Central retinal artery inclusion and high levels of acute intraocular hypertension are cell body, or gray matter, diseases. In a cell body disease, where the ganglion cell soma is affected, the cell metabolism is directly affected. The window for changing the outcome is low, that is, approximately 45 to 90 minutes for cell rescue. Therapies must be delivered rapidly after injury. In axonal injuries, the metabolism is affected indirectly, so the window of opportunity is longer and therapies can be delivered after the injury.

Most trials of neuroprotection have failed in diseases such as stroke and head trauma. However, neuroprotection trials have been successful in spinal cord trauma—an axonal disease—and in amyotrophic lateral sclerosis and Alzheimer's disease, both chronic neurodegenerative diseases. Glaucoma has features of both axonal and chronic disease and is therefore a good candidate for neuroprotection.

SUMMARY

In summary, glaucoma is primarily an anterior optic nerve disease and a chronic axonal disease. As with other axonal neuronal diseases, optic nerve diseases can be treated with neuroprotection. Glaucoma can be considered a very good candidate for neuroprotection.

REFERENCES

1. The AGIS Investigators. The advanced glaucoma intervention study, 6: effect of cataract on visual field and visual acuity. The AGIS Investigators. *Arch Ophthalmol* 2000;118:1639–1652.
2. The AGIS Investigators. The Advanced Glaucoma Intervention Study (AGIS): 1. Study design and methods and baseline characteristics of study patients. *Control Clin Trials* 1994;15:299–325.
3. Collaborative Normal-Tension Glaucoma Study Group. The effectiveness of intraocular pressure reduction in the treatment of

normal-tension glaucoma. Collaborative Normal-Tension Glaucoma Study Group. *Am J Ophthalmol* 1998;126:498–505.

4. Collaborative Normal-Tension Glaucoma Study Group. Comparison of glaucomatous progression between untreated patients with normal-tension glaucoma and patients with therapeutically reduced intraocular pressures. Collaborative Normal-Tension Glaucoma Study Group. *Am J Ophthalmol* 1998;126:487–497.

5. Lichter PR, Musch DC, Gillespie BW, et al. Interim clinical outcomes in the Collaborative Initial Glaucoma Treatment Study comparing initial treatment randomized to medications or surgery. *Ophthalmology* 2001;108:1943–1953.

6. Heijl A, Leske MC, Bengtsson B, et al. Reduction of intraocular pressure and glaucoma progression: results from the Early Manifest Glaucoma Trial. *Arch Ophthalmol* 2002;120:1268–1279.

7. Nouri-Mahdavi K, Hoffman D, Coleman AL, et al. Predictive factors for glaucomatous visual field progression in the Advanced Glaucoma Intervention Study. *Ophthalmology* 2004;111: 1627–1635.

8. Asrani S, Zeimer R, Wilensky J, et al. Large diurnal fluctuations in intraocular pressure are an independent risk factor in patients with glaucoma. *J Glaucoma* 2000;9:134–142.

9. Zeimer RC, Wilensky JT, Gieser DK, et al. Association between intraocular pressure peaks and progression of visual field loss. *Ophthalmology* 1991;98:64–69.

10. Burgoyne CF, Downs JC, Bellezza AJ, et al. The optic nerve head as a biomechanical structure: a new paradigm for understanding the role of IOP-related stress and strain in the pathophysiology of glaucomatous optic nerve head damage. *Prog Retin Eye Res* 2005;24:39–73.

11. Levin LA. Relevance of the site of injury of glaucoma to neuroprotective strategies. *Surv Ophthalmol* 2001;45(Suppl 3):S243–S249; discussion S273–S276.

12. Boden C, Sample PA, Boehm AG, et al. The structure-function relationship in eyes with glaucomatous visual field loss that crosses the horizontal meridian. *Arch Ophthalmol* 2002;120:907–912.

2

THE ROLE OF GLUTAMATE IN NEURODEGENERATIVE DISEASES INCLUDING GLAUCOMA

STUART A. LIPTON, MD, PHD

In glaucoma, as in many other neurodegenerative diseases, excessive stimulation of glutamate receptors is believed to occur. This article will provide a brief primer on the role of glutamate in a number of nervous system diseases, the rationale for targeting glutamate excitotoxicity with neuroprotective strategies, and the molecular mechanism of memantine, a neuroprotective agent that blocks glutamate excitotoxicity.

THE ROLE OF GLUTAMATE EXCITOTOXICITY IN NEUROLOGIC DISORDERS

Many neurologic disorders are mediated—at least in part—by overactivation of glutamate receptors (on both neurons and glia), which results in the influx of excessive Ca^{2+} through the receptors' associated ion channel, with subsequent free radical formation. Disorders in which excessive stimulation of glutamate receptors are thought to occur include focal cerebral ischemia; head and spinal cord trauma; epilepsy; Parkinson's disease; Alzheimer's disease; Huntington's disease; human immunodeficiency virus-associated dementia; amyotrophic lateral sclerosis; multiple sclerosis; glaucoma; mitochondrial disorders; metabolic disorders; neuropathic pain; drug addiction, tolerance, and withdrawal; depression; and possibly other psychiatric syndromes.

It is well known that glutamate is the major excitatory neuro-transmitter in the brain and that glutamate-mediated synaptic transmission is critical for the normal functioning of the nervous system. Most neurons, as well as glial cells, contain high concentrations of glutamate. However, if neurons or the supporting glial are injured and unable to properly control the regulation or clearance of glutamate, secondary damage can result—even if the primary cause of the disease has nothing to do with glutamate. Injured neurons become exquisitely vulnerable to even normal levels of glutamate. This overstimulation by glutamate can literally excite cells to death. John Olney coined the term "excitotoxicity" to describe this phenomenon.[1] We have known since 1957 that excitotoxicity occurs in retinal ganglion cells.[2]

There are various types of glutamate receptors. The one most prominently involved in neuronal damage is the N-methyl-D-aspartate (NMDA)-type glutamate receptor. When activated, the NMDA receptor opens a channel that allows Ca^{2+} and other cations to move into the cell (Fig. 2-1). Under normal conditions of synaptic transmission, the NMDA receptor is activated for only brief periods of time (milliseconds). Under pathologic conditions, however, overactivation of the receptor for longer periods causes excessive influx of Ca^{2+} into the nerve cell, which then triggers a variety of biochemical processes that can lead to dendritic and synaptic damage, and even to neuronal cell death. Excess influx of Ca^{2+} can overload the mitochondria, the energy storehouses of the cell, resulting in oxygen free radical formation, activation of caspase, and release of apoptosis-inducing factor.[3] The Ca^{2+} coming into neurons through NMDA receptor-associated channels can also activate neuronal nitric oxide synthase (NOS),[4] leading to increased nitric oxide (NO) production and the formation of toxic peroxynitrite ($ONOO^-$) when NO reacts with superoxide anion (O_2^-).[5] Peroxynitrite causes significant damage to the cell. Also, stimulation of mitogen-activated protein kinases (including p38 mitogen-activated protein kinase) activates transcription factors (e.g., myocyte-enhancer factor 2C or MEF2C) that can enter the nucleus to influence neuronal injury and apoptosis (an energy-requiring form of cell death that usually involves condensation of the nucleus and DNA fragmentation). Recently, we discovered an extracellular pathway in which NO traverses the cell and activates matrix metalloproteinases, enzymes that destroy the extracellular

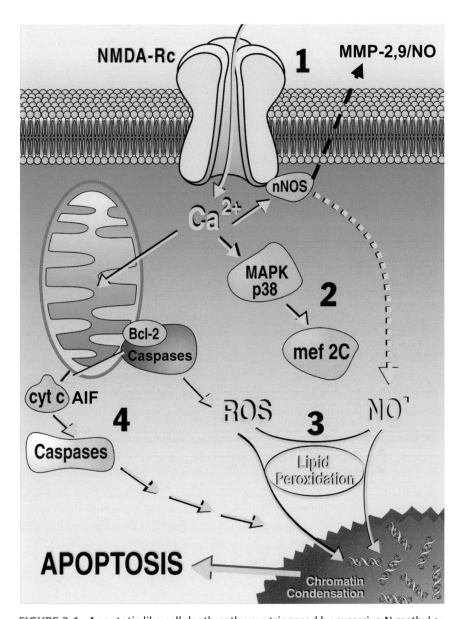

FIGURE 2-1. Apoptotic-like cell death pathways triggered by excessive N-methyl-D-aspartate (NMDA) receptor activity. The cascade of steps leading to neuronal cell death include the following: (1) NMDA receptor hyperactivation; (2) activation of the p38 mitogen-activated protein kinase–MEF2C (transcription factor) pathway (MEF2C is subsequently cleaved by caspase to form an endogenous dominant-interfering form that contributes to neuronal cell death); (3) toxic effects of free radicals such as nitric oxide (NO) and reactive oxygen species (ROS); and (4) mitochondrial-mediated activation of enzymes, including caspase and apoptosis-inducing factor, that lead to neuronal injury and apoptosis. nNOS, nitric oxide synthase; cyt c, cytochrome c. (Source: Lipton SA. Paradigm shift in NMDA receptor antagonist drug development: molecular mechanism of uncompetitive inhibition by memantine in the treatment of Alzheimer's disease and other neurologic disorders. *J Alzheimer's Dis* 2004;6:S61–S74.)

matrix located outside of the cell. This destruction of extracellular matrix can lead to neuronal cell death because cells lose contact with their neighbors (a form of apoptosis known as anoikis).

Because excessive glutamate receptor activation attacks the cell in so many ways, there are many potential targets for neuroprotection. However, it has been very difficult to develop neuroprotective drugs that are also clinically tolerated to ameliorate insults to the retina and other areas of the brain. A clinically acceptable antiexcitotoxic therapy must be able to block excessive activation of the NMDA receptor while leaving normal function relatively intact. To date, our group has shown that three clinically tolerated drugs can be potentially used for neuroprotection. Only one of these drugs, memantine, acts on the NMDA-type glutamate receptor and has been shown to be clinically tolerated in humans at neuroprotective concentrations. In addition, nitroglycerin can potentially be targeted to the NMDA receptor to work safely. Finally, the antianemia drug, erythropoietin, can act downstream from the NMDA receptor to ameliorate neurotoxicity. Because of their proven safety record, these drugs, or new derivatives of them, can be tested in clinical trials relatively quickly.

CHARACTERIZING THE GLUTAMATE RECEPTOR

Our laboratory has cloned and characterized various brain receptors, including novel subunits of the NMDA receptor. NMDA is not an endogenous substance in the body; it is an experimental tool that is highly selective for this subtype of glutamate receptor.[6,7]

Classic NMDA receptors consist of two types of subunits (NR1 and NR2A-D) with binding sites for glutamate, the endogenous agonist, and for glycine, a co-agonist for receptor activation (Fig. 2-2). In addition, some NMDA receptors have NR3A or B subunits. To use an analogy to describe its function, the NMDA receptor can be thought of as a television set—with an on/off switch and a volume control. The agonist sites are similar to the on/off switch. Drugs developed to block the agonist sites are called "competitive antagonists" because they compete one-to-one with glycine or glutamate. Thus, as the concentration of these drugs is increased, they block lower, normal levels of glutamate before blocking pathologically high levels, and thus block the normal

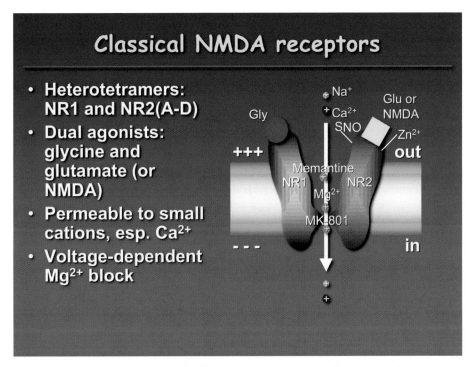

FIGURE 2-2. NMDA receptor model illustrating important binding and modulatory sites. Glu or NMDA: glutamate or NMDA binding site. Gly: glycine binding site. Zn^{2+}: zinc binding site. NR1: NMDA receptor subunit 1. NR2: NMDA receptor subunit 2A. SNO: cysteine sulfhydryl group (-SH) reacting with nitric oxide species (NO). X: Mg^{2+}, MK-801, and memantine binding sites within the ion channel pore region. (Source: Lipton SA. Paradigm shift in NMDA receptor antagonist drug development: molecular mechanism of uncompetitive inhibition by memantine in the treatment of Alzheimer's disease and other neurologic disorders. *J Alzheimer's Dis* 2004;6:S61–S74.)

functioning of the neuron before blocking the pathologic function, resulting in side effects. This strategy, therefore, does not work in treating neurologic disorders, as demonstrated in many Phase III clinical trials.

So, to continue with the television analogy, we need to find the equivalent of the volume control of the NMDA receptor—or the "gain of the receptor." When excessive Ca^{2+} fluxes through the NMDA receptor-associated ion channel, this is similar to the volume being too loud, and we would want to turn down the "volume" of the flux toward normal. Because the NMDA receptor is a very fancy television set, it has several volume knobs, one of which relates to Mg^{2+} binding in the ion channel. However, Mg^{2+} block is a "flickery block" and does not effectively compete with excessive Ca^{2+} influx. Although Mg^{2+} affects the right site, it does not turn the volume down far enough.

Turning the volume all the way down would be equivalent to turning off the "on/off" switch in terms of blocking normal functioning of the television. This is the case with a drug called dizocilpine or MK-801. Although MK-801 is a very good excitotoxicity blocker, the drug has a very long "dwell time" in the ion channel—reflecting its slow "off-rate"—and therefore accumulates in the channels to block neurotransmission and thus critical normal functions. Other drugs with slightly shorter but still excessive dwell times can lead to hallucinations (e.g., phencyclidine, or "Angel Dust") or drowsiness (e.g., ketamine, a Food and Drug Administration-approved anesthetic).

MEMANTINE

A clinically tolerated NMDA receptor antagonist would block excessive NMDA receptor activation while sparing normal neurotransmission, and would not cause drowsiness or hallucinations. Such a drug would have a slower "off-rate" than Mg^{2+} and a faster off-rate than MK-801, and would block NMDA receptor-operated channels only when they are excessively open. Results from our experiments have suggested that memantine is such a drug.

Memantine, a derivative of the antiviral drug amantadine, was first synthesized by Eli Lilly and Company and patented in 1968. The reported efficacy of amantadine (and therefore potentially memantine) in Parkinson's disease was discovered by serendipity in a patient taking amantadine for influenza, and led scientists to believe that the compounds were dopaminergic or anticholinergic (which we later found to be incorrect at clinically tolerated concentrations).

Memantine has a three-ring structure with a bridgehead amine that normally carries a positive charge ($-NH^{3+}$) and binds at or near the Mg^{2+} site in the NMDA receptor-associated channel (Fig. 2-3). Unlike amantadine, memantine has two methyl (-CH) side groups that prolong its dwell time in the channel and make it a much better NMDA channel blocker than amantadine. Research at Merz (Frankfurt, Germany) suggested that the drug could block NMDA currents in a potent fashion, but we subse-

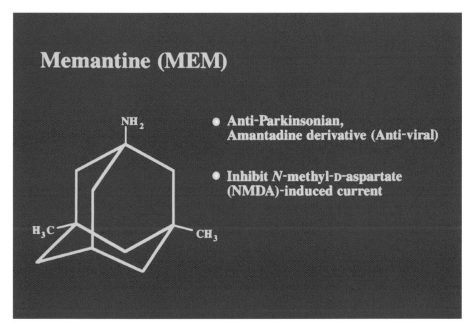

FIGURE 2-3. Chemical structure of memantine. (Source: Lipton SA. Paradigm shift in NMDA receptor antagonist drug development: molecular mechanism of uncompetitive inhibition by memantine in the treatment of Alzheimer's disease and other neurologic disorders. *J Alzheimer's Dis* 2004;6:S61–S74.)

quently found that memantine was, in fact, a rather impotent blocker of NMDA channels but did so in a unique pharmacologic fashion that could be harnessed clinically.

The blockade of NMDA-induced ionic currents by memantine is illustrated in Figure 2-4. In a sample experiment, the membrane voltage of a neuron was held at the resting potential. The application of 12 μM memantine produced an effective blockade only during NMDA receptor activation. (This concentration of memantine is similar to the level of 1–12 μM that can be achieved in the human brain when the drug is used for Parkinson's disease.) When the memantine application was stopped, the NMDA response returned to previous levels over a period of approximately 5 seconds. So, memantine obviously blocked the current, and then washed out relatively quickly—although not immediately as with Mg^{2+}. The other antagonist discussed earlier, MK-801, would virtually never wash out under these conditions. The findings indicate that memantine is

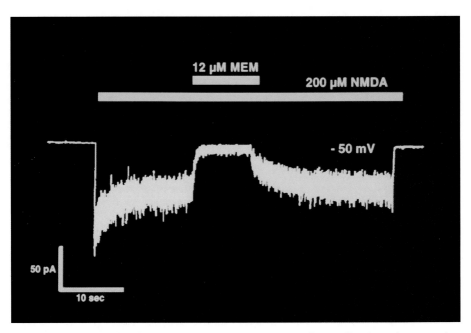

FIGURE 2-4. Blockade of NMDA current by memantine. The application of memantine produced an effective blockade only during NMDA receptor activation, consistent with the notion that its mechanism of action is open-channel block. (Source: Lipton SA. Paradigm shift in NMDA receptor antagonist drug development: molecular mechanism of uncompetitive inhibition by memantine in the treatment of Alzheimer's disease and other neurologic disorders. *J Alzheimer's Dis* 2004;6:S61–S74.)

an effective, but temporary, NMDA receptor blocker and has the right kinetic signature for safety.

Although Big Pharma has traditionally developed drugs by high-affinity screening, in point of fact, high affinity can lead to severe side effects because of blockade of normal target function. Under physiologic conditions, the affinity of memantine for the NMDA receptor is very low, that is, in the micromolar range. Initially, this finding led researchers to consider memantine a poor candidate for neuroprotection. However, affinity should not be confused with selectivity. High affinity per se is not the key issue, as long as a drug acts selectively and specifically on the target of interest, and the effective concentration can be achieved. Memantine, at a micromolar concentration, is quite selective for the NMDA-type channel.

Another experiment showed that memantine was relatively ineffective at blocking low levels of receptor activity (i.e., those associated with normal synaptic activity and neurologic function), but became very effective at higher concentrations[8,9] (Fig. 2-5). This effect is a classic example of "uncompetitive" antagonism, meaning that (at a fixed dose) a drug inhibits better when there is more, rather than less, agonist.

The favorable clinical safety profile seen to date with memantine can be explained by the pharmacokinetics of its action in the NMDA receptor-associated ion channel. Memantine preferen-

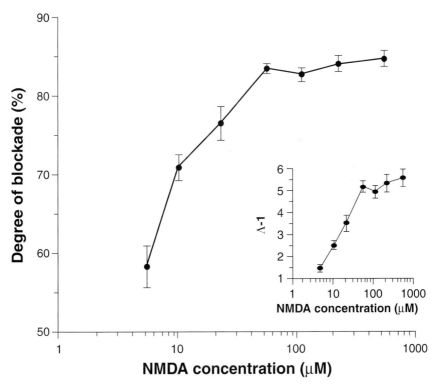

FIGURE 2-5. Memantine's "uncompetitive antagonism." Paradoxically, a fixed dose of memantine (i.e., 1 μM) blocks the effect of increasing concentrations of NMDA to a greater degree than lower concentrations of NMDA. (Source: Lipton SA. Paradigm shift in NMDA receptor antagonist drug development: molecular mechanism of uncompetitive inhibition by memantine in the treatment of Alzheimer's disease and other neurologic disorders. *J Alzheimer's Dis* 2004;6:S61–S74.)

tially blocks NMDA receptor activity if the ion channel is excessively open, that is, when there is more glutamate. This is known as "open-channel block." When there is more glutamate, more channels open because of receptor activation, and memantine is more effective at entering the channels and blocking them. Thus, memantine essentially acts only under pathologic conditions, and relatively spares normal activity when the channels are opening and closing normally (Fig. 2-6).

Most importantly, unlike MK-801, memantine does not accumulate in the channels, blocking neurotransmission (Fig. 2-7). Memantine only blocks approximately 15% of normal neurotransmission, which explains its safety.

Memantine has been shown to protect retinal ganglion cells from death[9,10] (Fig. 2-8). Memantine has also been shown to provide protection against stroke and can be given up to 2 hours after a stroke.[10]

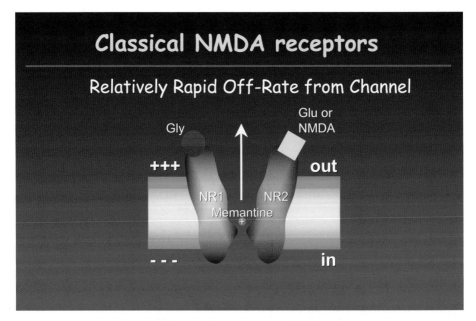

FIGURE 2-6. Memantine preferentially enters the NMDA receptor-operated channel when there is excessive activity. As soon as the "volume" is turned back down (i.e., there is less influx of Ca^{2+}), memantine comes back out of the channel, and thus has a relatively rapid "off-rate."

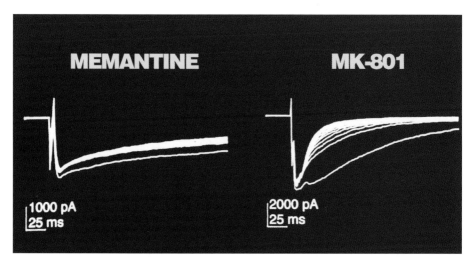

FIGURE 2-7. Memantine relatively spares normal neurotransmission. MK-801 blocks all of the NMDA current in the synapse and accumulates in the channels. Memantine 1 μM only blocks approximately 15% of normal neural transmission. Note that the initial segment of excitatory synaptic activity is mediated by another type of glutamate receptor, the AMPA receptor, and is not blocked by memantine or MK-801. The second half of the trace is mediated by NMDA receptors. MK-801 exhibits use dependence and progressively blocks all NMDA activity, whereas memantine blocks relatively little NMDA activity under physiologic conditions. (Source: Chen H-SV, Wang YF, Rayudu PV, et al. Neuroprotective concentrations of the N-methyl-D-aspartate open-channel blocker memantine are effective without cytoplasmic vacuolation following post-ischemic administration and do not block maze learning or long-term potentiation. *Neuroscience* 1998;86:1121–1132.)

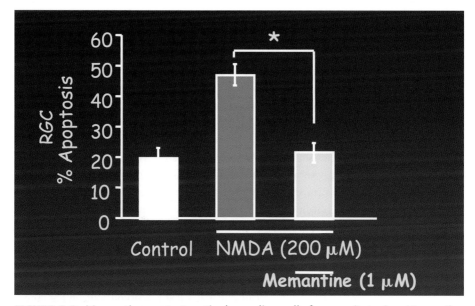

FIGURE 2-8. Memantine protects retinal ganglion cells from excitotoxins. Memantine (1 μM) blocks apoptosis of retinal ganglion cells induced by exposure to NMDA. (Source: S.A. Lipton, unpublished data.)

TABLE 2-1. CLINICAL TRIALS WITH MEMANTINE[11–17]

Trial	Result
German/Merz Phase III trial for vascular dementia and Alzheimer's disease	+
Karolinska/Italian Phase III trial for vascular dementia	+
Three U.S. multicenter Phase III trials for Alzheimer's disease	+
United Kingdom Phase III trial for vascular dementia	+
French Phase III trial for vascular dementia	+
U.S. Phase II trial for diabetic neuropathic pain	+/−
U.S. Phase II trial for HIV-associated dementia	+/−

HIV, human immunodeficiency virus.

A series of human clinical trials have been launched to investigate the efficacy of memantine in the treatment of Alzheimer's disease, vascular dementia, human immunodeficiency virus-associated dementia, diabetic neuropathic pain, and depression, as well as glaucoma (Table 2-1). The efficacy of memantine demonstrated in these trials to date suggests that memantine, and drugs acting in a similar manner, could become important new weapons in the fight against neuronal damage.

SUMMARY

In summary, apoptosis-mediated excitotoxic cell death is implicated in the pathophysiology of many neurologic diseases, including glaucoma. This excitotoxicity is caused, at least in part, by excessive activation of NMDA-type glutamate receptors. Although blockade of NMDA receptor activity prevents excitotoxicity, only those NMDA blockers that selectively reduce excessive receptor activation without affecting normal function will be clinically tolerated. Memantine, a neuroprotective agent that blocks excessive NMDA receptor activation, but not normal activation, was recently approved by the Food and Drug Administration for the treatment of Alzheimer's disease and is also used in Europe for vascular dementia. We have shown that memantine is an uncompetitive, open-channel blocker with a fast off-rate; as such, it blocks excessive NMDA receptor activity while relatively sparing normal activity. Further clinical studies on the efficacy of memantine in the treatment of glaucoma and other neurodegenerative diseases are currently under way.

REFERENCES

1. Olney JW. Glutamate-induced retinal degeneration in neonatal mice. Electron microscopy of the acutely evolving lesion. *J Neuropathol Exp Neurol* 1969;28:455–474.
2. Lucas DR, Newhouse JP. The toxic effect of sodium L-glutamate on the inner layers of the retina. *AMA Arch Ophthalmol* 1957; 58:193–201.
3. Budd SL, Tenneti L, Lishnak T, et al. Mitochondrial and extramitochondrial apoptotic signaling pathways in cerebrocortical neurons. *Proc Natl Acad Sci U S A* 2000;97:6161–6166.
4. Dawson VL, Dawson TM, London ED, et al. Nitric oxide mediates glutamate neurotoxicity in primary cortical cultures. *Proc Natl Acad Sci U S A* 1991;88:6368–6371.
5. Lipton SA, Choi Y-B, Pan ZH, et al. A redox-based mechanism for the neuroprotective and neurodestructive effects of nitric oxide and related nitroso-compounds. *Nature* 1993;364:626–632.
6. Lipton SA. Erythropoietin for neurologic protection and diabetic neuropathy. *N Engl J Med* 2004;350:2516–2517.
7. Lipton SA. Turning down, but not off. *Nature* 2004;428:473.
8. Lipton SA. Prospects for clinically tolerated NMDA antagonists: open-channel blockers and alternative redox states of nitric oxide. *Trends Neurosci* 1993;16:527–532.
9. Chen H-SV, Pellegrini JW, Aggarwal SK, et al. Open-channel block of N-methyl-D-aspartate (NMDA) responses by memantine: therapeutic advantage against NMDA receptor-mediated neurotoxicity. *J Neurosci* 1992;12:4427–4436.
10. Chen H-SV, Wang YF, Rayudu PV, et al. Neuroprotective concentrations of the N-methyl-D-aspartate open-channel blocker memantine are effective without cytoplasmic vacuolation following post-ischemic administration and do not block maze learning or long-term potentiation. *Neuroscience* 1998;86:1121–1132.
11. Lipton SA. Paradigm shift in NMDA receptor antagonist drug development: molecular mechanism of uncompetitive inhibition by memantine in the treatment of Alzheimer's disease and other neurologic disorders. *J Alzheimer's Dis* 2004;6:S61–S74.
12. Winblad B, Poritis N. Memantine in severe dementia: results of the 9M-Best Study (benefit and efficacy in severely demented patients during treatment with memantine). *Int J Geriatr Psychiatry* 1999;14:135–146.
13. Wilcock G, Mobius HJ, Stoffler A. A double-blind, placebo-controlled multicentre study of memantine in mild to moderate vascular dementia (MMM500). *Int Clin Psychopharmacol* 2002;17:297–305.

14. Reisberg B, Doody R, Stoffler A, et al. Memantine in moderate-to-severe Alzheimer's disease. *N Engl J Med* 2003;348:1333–1341.

15. Tariot PN, Farlow MR, Grossberg GT, et al. Memantine treatment in patients with moderate to severe Alzheimer disease already receiving donepezil: a randomized controlled trial. *JAMA* 2004;291:317–324.

16. Orgogozo JM, Rigaud AS, Stoffler A, et al. Efficacy and safety of memantine in patients with mild to moderate vascular dementia: a randomized, placebo-controlled trial (MMM 300). *Stroke* 2002;33:1834–1839.

17. Le DA, Lipton SA. Potential and current use of N-methyl-D-aspartate (NMDA) receptor antagonists in diseases of aging. *Drugs Aging* 2001;18:717–724.

3

NEUROPROTECTION WITH MEMANTINE IN ALZHEIMER'S DISEASE: WHAT IS THE CLINICAL EVIDENCE?

LUTZ FRÖLICH, MD, PHD

Alzheimer's disease, like glaucoma, is a chronic and degenerative disease with a very long latency period. Disease progress occurs years before symptoms appear (Fig. 3-1). One of the core symptoms of Alzheimer's disease is the decline in cognitive performance—learning, memory, and associated cognitive functions. However, these symptoms appear late during the disease process, whereas other noncognitive symptoms, for example, apathy and depressive mood, may appear earlier, but are nonspecific and difficult to quantify.

Obviously, clinical trials with antidementia drugs must take into account the relevant clinical symptomatology and show efficacy on these levels. Several randomized clinical trials have demonstrated significant improvements in patients receiving memantine for vascular dementia and Alzheimer's disease[1–4] over placebo, and these are summarized in Table 3-1.

In the following chapter, the clinical data on memantine in Alzheimer's disease will be analyzed in detail in terms of whether they demonstrate neuroprotection on a clinical level.

EFFICACY OF MEMANTINE IN ALZHEIMER'S DISEASE

The efficacy of memantine in Alzheimer's disease was demonstrated in a placebo-controlled double-blind study by Reisberg et

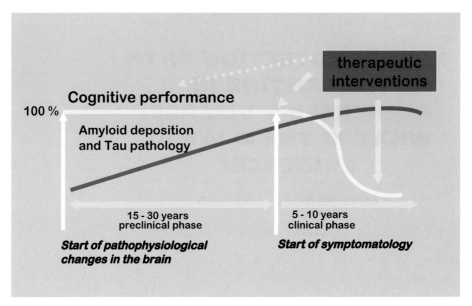

FIGURE 3-1. Neuroprotective approaches in Alzheimer's disease: problems of present clinical studies.

TABLE 3-1. RECENT CLINICAL STUDIES WITH MEMANTINE IN DEMENTIA

	Sample size	Duration of study	Degree of dementia	Trial outcome (variables in favor of memantine)
Wilcock et al.[1]	548	6 mo	Mild to moderate	Significant improvement in cognitive functions
Orgogozo et al.[2]	288	6 mo	Mild to moderate	Significant improvement in cognitive functions
Winblad and Poritis[3]	166	3 mo	Severe	Significant improvement —motor functions —cognitive disturbances —social behavior
Reisberg et al.[4]	252	6 mo	Moderate to severe	Significant improvement —cognition —activities of daily living —global assessment

al.,[4] which was the basis for the U.S. Food and Drug Administration approval of memantine for the treatment of moderate-to-severe forms of the disease. In this study, 250 patients with moderate-to-severe Alzheimer's disease were randomly assigned to receive placebo or 20 mg of memantine daily for 28 weeks, an appropriate minimal timeline for a clinical study in Alzheimer's disease. Treatment differences between baseline and end point were assessed using standard measures of cognition, function, and behavior.

The results showed better clinical outcomes for patients in the treatment group versus the placebo group. The treatment group had significant improvements in scores for the Severe Impairment Battery (SIB), a test that evaluates cognitive performance in advanced Alzheimer's disease (Fig. 3-2). However, because Alzheimer's disease extends beyond cognitive symptoms, it is also important to assess function when evaluating the clinically meaningful effects of a treatment. In this study, patients in the memantine group scored better than the placebo group in their ability to

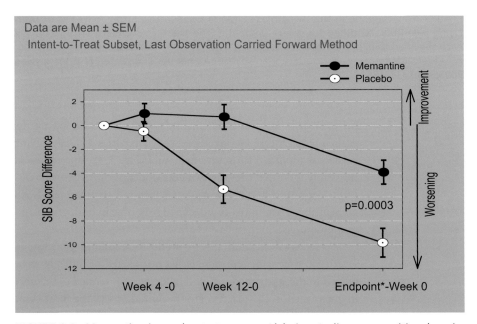

FIGURE 3-2. Memantine in moderate-to-severe Alzheimer's disease: cognitive domain. Change from baseline in Severe Impairment Battery (SIB) scores. The mean (± standard error) scores at each specified time in the observed-cases analysis. (Source: Reisberg B, Doody R, Stoffler A, et al. Memantine in moderate-to-severe Alzheimer's disease. *N Engl J Med* 2003;348:1333–1341.)

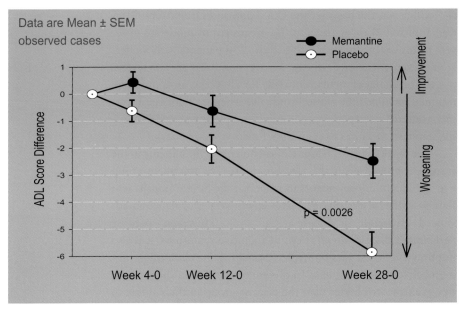

FIGURE 3-3. Memantine in moderate-to-severe Alzheimer's disease: functional domain. Change from baseline in the Alzheimer's Disease Cooperative Study Activities of Daily Living Inventory, modified for severe dementia. The mean (± standard error) scores at each specified time in the observed cases analysis. (Source: Reisberg B, Doody R, Stoffler A, et al. Memantine in moderate-to-severe Alzheimer's disease. *N Engl J Med* 2003;348:1333–1341.)

perform daily tasks and remain independent, as assessed by the Alzheimer's Disease Cooperative Study Activities of Daily Living Inventory modified for severe dementia (Fig. 3-3). The results of this study indicated that the two core domains of Alzheimer's disease—cognition and function—can respond to treatment with memantine. These functions declined over time in both groups, although more so in the placebo group.

As far as safety, most adverse events were mild to moderate in severity in this study and were either not related or unlikely to be related to the study medication. Hallucinations tended to be more frequent than in the placebo group. Agitation was the most common reason for discontinuation of treatment in this study and was more common in the placebo group.

Since publication of the Reisberg et al.[4] study, a number of other studies have been carried out on the effects of memantine in Alzheimer's disease. A study by Tariot et al.[5] showed a very interesting phenomenon in patients receiving a cholinesterase inhibitor. In this randomized, double-blind, placebo-controlled clinical trial, the efficacy and safety of memantine versus placebo were evaluated in 404 patients with moderate-to-severe Alzheimer's disease who were already receiving stable treatment with donepezil. Participants were randomized to receive add-on treatment with memantine (starting dose 5 mg/day, increased to 20 mg/day, n = 203) or placebo (n = 201) for 24 weeks.

The results showed that memantine resulted in significantly better outcomes than placebo on measures of cognition, activities of daily living, global outcome, and behavior. Mean change from baseline by visit and at end point on the SIB showed statistically significant differences between the memantine and placebo groups at all visits beginning at week 8; the mean SIB values for the patients receiving memantine remained above baseline throughout the trial (Fig. 3-4).

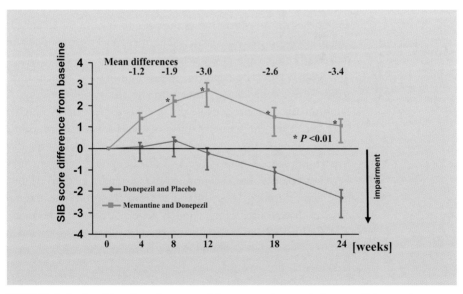

FIGURE 3-4. Combination therapy with memantine and donepezil in moderate-to-severe Alzheimer's disease. Mean change from baseline by visit and at end point on the SIB by using observed case and last observation carried forward, showing statistically significant differences between the memantine and placebo groups at all visits beginning at week 8; the mean SIB values for the patients receiving memantine remained above baseline throughout the trial. (Source: Tariot PN, Farlow MR, Grossberg GT, et al. Memantine treatment in patients with moderate to severe Alzheimer disease already receiving donepezil: a randomized controlled trial. *JAMA* 2004;291:317–324.)

This controlled trial demonstrated that in patients with moderate-to-severe Alzheimer's disease, those who received add-on therapy with memantine performed significantly better after 24 weeks than those who just continued with their previous donepezil therapy. This combination of memantine with cholinesterase inhibitor, with their different mechanisms of action, may become an appropriate and effective therapy.

NEUROPROTECTION IN ALZHEIMER'S DISEASE?

One of the principal difficulties in assessing neuroprotection in Alzheimer's disease is that a half-year controlled trial situation is only a small fragment of the natural disease course. Alzheimer's disease is a chronic disease with at least 7 to 10 years of natural cause. Thus, the pivotal trials with antidementia drugs have always been extended over 1 to 5 years of continuous treatment. After the end of the controlled trial, all of the patients (i.e., in the treatment and placebo groups) were switched to open-label treatment and an untreated comparison group was lacking.

From a clinical perspective, the demonstration of neuroprotective effect depends very much on the efficacy of the drug. A symptomatic drug may enable the patients to perform at a higher level, and then the natural course of the disease may continue. With a strong-acting, symptomatic drug, this can make a big difference initially. A neuroprotective disease-modifying agent may have less potency, but if continued over extended periods of time may demonstrate a large difference from the projected, natural cause of disease after a long enough period of time. Furthermore, if clinical performance remains on the same level for an extended period of time after stopping drug treatment as it was with drug treatment, this would also be taken as an indication for neuroprotection.

So in principle, the answer to the question of whether there is neuroprotection with memantine in Alzheimer's disease depends strongly on the timeframe of the study course and on the extent of the drug's actual effects on symptoms. Both the shift in slope and the demonstration of clinical efficacy after stopping the drug may indicate neuroprotection. Several modifications in the design of clinical trials may help to answer this question, but they require long-term studies of more than 1 year and/or large patient samples, for example, staggered start or randomized withdrawal, inclusion of biomarkers, functional end points in long-term observational trials, and long-term investigations of populations at risk. Such studies have not been performed with memantine.

In the extension studies with memantine, as with all other presently available antidementive agents, all patients' conditions worsen compared with their baseline after a 1-year period. However, because of the lack of a placebo group, the slope of decline in these patients cannot really be compared with the natural course of disease. The question then remains: Is the slope of decline, which can be observed under memantine in the extension studies, different from the slope of decline under the natural course of disease?

Another way that clinical researchers have attempted to study neuroprotection is to measure synaptic activity using biologic markers such as cerebral glucose metabolism. A pilot study by Potkin[6] used positron emission tomography imaging to measure the effect of memantine (10 mg twice per day) on regional cerebral glucose metabolism in 10 patients with mild-to-moderate Alzheimer's disease. After 24 weeks, patients who received memantine in this randomized, placebo-controlled, double-blind study showed a statistically significant increase in glucose metabolism in several regions of the brain associated with language and attention. In contrast, placebo-treated patients showed metabolic declines in several of these same regions. Although these data were from a small number of patients and need to be confirmed in larger scale studies, they indicate the potential for neuroprotection with memantine.

SUMMARY

Neuroprotection in central nervous system disorders is a concept primarily derived from experimental studies and is actually difficult to prove in clinical trials. The convincing preclinical evidence of the neuroprotective potential of memantine in Alzheimer's disease has not been fully transformed into clinical evidence (i.e., modification of disease progression). Additional clinical trials are needed that may incorporate, for example, staggered start or randomized withdrawal designs, inclusion of biomarkers, functional end points in long-term observational trials, or long-term investigations of populations at risk. However, among the currently available drugs for dementias, memantine has the best potential to show neuroprotection in the clinical situation.

REFERENCES

1. Wilcock G, Mobius HJ, Stoffler A. A double-blind, placebo-controlled multicentre study of memantine in mild to moderate vascular dementia (MMM500). *Int Clin Psychopharmacol* 2002; 17:297–305.
2. Orgogozo JM, Rigaud AS, Stoffler A, et al. Efficacy and safety of memantine in patients with mild to moderate vascular dementia: a randomized, placebo-controlled trial (MMM 300). *Stroke* 2002;33:1834–1839.
3. Winblad B, Poritis N. Memantine in severe dementia: results of the 9M-Best Study (Benefit and efficacy in severely demented patients during treatment with memantine). *Int J Geriatr Psychiatry* 1999;14:135–146.
4. Reisberg B, Doody R, Stoffler A, et al. Memantine in moderate-to-severe Alzheimer's disease. *N Engl J Med* 2003;348:1333–1341.
5. Tariot PN, Farlow MR, Grossberg GT, et al. Memantine treatment in patients with moderate to severe Alzheimer disease already receiving donepezil: a randomized controlled trial. *JAMA* 2004;291:317–324.
6. Potkin SG. Namenda (memantine) appears to produce positive effect on brain activity in patients with mild to moderate Alzheimer's disease. American Academy of Neurology Annual Meeting, San Francisco, 2004.

4

RATIONALE FOR MEMANTINE IN THE TREATMENT OF GLAUCOMA: PRECLINICAL DATA

WILLIAM HARE, OD, PHD, ELIZABETH WOLDEMUSSIE, PHD, AND LARRY WHEELER, PHD

Glutamate is the principle excitatory transmitter in the central nervous system (CNS), including the retina. Excessive activation of glutamate receptors is injurious to neurons and may be involved in a wide range of neurodegenerative disorders. Elevated levels of retinal extracellular glutamate have been reported in experimental models of retinal disease including glaucoma.

In the retina, glutamate is released by photoreceptors, bipolar cells, and ganglion cells (Fig. 4-1). In fact, the density of N-methyl-D-aspartate (NMDA)-type glutamatergic receptors is probably greatest in retinal ganglion cells (RGCs). It has been shown that overactivation of NMDA-type glutamate receptors contributes significantly to "excitotoxic" injury of RGCs resulting from a wide range of insults in animal models. Overactivation of NMDA receptors may result from accumulation of glutamate in the extracellular space but can also occur in the presence of normal extracellular glutamate levels if the neuronal cell has been otherwise injured or metabolically compromised. In models of both acute and chronic injury to the retina and optic nerve, evidence for glutamate dysregulation has been determined either directly through microdialysis measures of extracellular glutamate concentration or indirectly through measured alterations in glutamate-buffering mechanisms

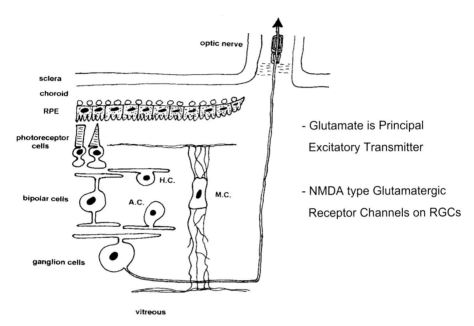

- Glutamate is Principal
  Excitatory Transmitter

- NMDA type Glutamatergic
  Receptor Channels on RGCs

FIGURE 4-1. Retina and optic nerve.

such as glutamate transporters. Because glaucomatous vision loss is the direct consequence of injury to RGCs, the RGC is the target cell for glaucomatous neuroprotection.

Treatment with memantine, a selective blocker of the NMDA-type glutamatergic ion channel, has been shown to prevent or reduce neuronal injury in a wide rage of animal models for CNS injury (Table 4-1). The unique properties of memantine binding within the glutamate channel result in a preferential block of excessive (excitotoxic) levels of glutamatergic activity with rela-

TABLE 4-1. MEMANTINE TREATMENT HAS BEEN SHOWN TO BE PROTECTIVE IN ANIMAL MODELS OF CENTRAL NERVOUS SYSTEM INJURY

- Cerebral ischemia (rat)
- Traumatic brain injury (rat)
- Alzheimer's disease (rat, mouse)
- Acute retina ischemia (rat and rabbit)
- Optic nerve ischemia (rabbit)
- Traumatic optic nerve injury (rat)
- Spontaneous glaucoma (DBA/2J mouse)
- Chronic experimental glaucoma (rat and monkey)

tively less effect on normal glutamatergic signaling. Thus, memantine treatment may be effective to reduce neuronal injury at concentrations (plasma levels) that have little or no effect on normal CNS function. In the following sections, results from studies using models of experimental glaucoma in the rat and monkey are summarized. The results show that memantine treatment is associated with a reduction of RGC injury in these models.

RAT EXPERIMENTAL GLAUCOMA MODEL

In an experimental glaucoma rat model developed by Wolde-Mussie et al.,[1] laser cautery of the episcleral and perilimbal veins was used to induce chronic ocular hypertension (COHT) and RGC injury. Laser treatment is followed by an increase in intraocular pressure (IOP) from approximately 15 mm Hg to approximately 30 mm Hg and is maintained at this higher level for at least 2 months. Histologic analysis of retinas from this model has shown that there is a progressive loss of RGCs with approximately 40% of the RGCs lost by 3 weeks after IOP elevation.

Test groups of animals were dosed at either 5 or 10 mg/kg per day using continuous administration with subcutaneous osmotic pumps. Dosing began immediately after laser treatment and lasted for 3 weeks, at which time the animals were sacrificed for histologic measures of RGC survival. The results summarized in Figure 4-2 show that the 5-mg dose was associated with a trend toward increased RGC survival (reduced loss), although this was not statistically significant. The 10-mg dose, however, was associated with a highly significant reduction of RGC loss to approximately 12%. In a separate experiment, the 10-mg dosing regimen was begun at 10 days after laser treatment, at a time when significant RGC loss is already evident in this model. Initiation of memantine treatment at this point was associated with an almost complete prevention of any further RGC loss (data not shown).

MONKEY EXPERIMENTAL GLAUCOMA MODEL

The efficacy and safety of memantine treatment were also evaluated in a monkey model for experimental glaucoma. We previously

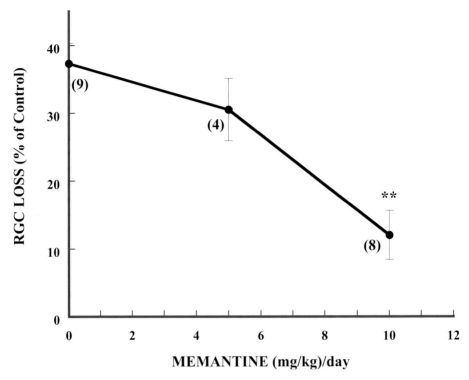

FIGURE 4-2. Memantine treatment reduces retinal ganglion cell (RGC) loss associated with experimental glaucoma in rat. Numbers in parentheses indicate the number of rats used for each dose. Values represent mean ± standard error of mean. (Source: Wolde-Mussie E, Yoles E, Schwartz M, et al. Neuroprotective effect of memantine in different retinal injury models in rats. *J Glaucoma* 2002;11:474–480.)

showed that memantine treatment is not associated with any significant effect on IOP in this model (data not shown). The methodology and results of this study are described in great detail in two recently published reports.[2,3] In this model, COHT was induced using a method originally described by Gaasterland and Kupfer.[4] Using a gonio-lens, argon laser energy was directed to the trabecular meshwork of the aqueous outflow tissue at the anterior chamber angle. This model has been used in many studies of glaucomatous injury to the retina and optic nerve.

In the study described here, 18 cynomolgus monkeys were divided into two treatment groups of 9 animals each. One group received daily oral dosing of 4 mg/kg memantine plus vehicle, whereas the other group received daily oral dosing with vehicle only. During a period of 16 months after laser treatment and IOP elevation, a battery of functional and structural assays was performed to evaluate the integrity of the retina and optic nerve. Functional measures included electroretinography (ERG) recordings using both conventional and multifocal methods, made at approximately 3, 5, and 16 months after IOP elevation. Recordings of the visually evoked cortical potential (VECP) were also made at 16 months. Structural assays included stereo fundus photos of the optic nerve head, retinal vessels, and peripapillary retina, taken at multiple time points during the study. Measures of optic nerve head topography were obtained from confocal laser scans (Heidelberg Retinal Tomograph; Heidelberg Engineering, Heidelberg, Germany) made at 3, 5, and 10 months after IOP elevation. At approximately 16 months, all animals were sacrificed and histologic counts of cells in the retinal RGC layer were made.

In all laser-treated eyes, laser treatment was followed rapidly by an increase in IOP to some peak level. In some eyes, IOP remained at a high level during the following 16 months, whereas it decreased to a somewhat lower level in other eyes. Figure 4-3 shows that both the peak IOP and subsequent IOP levels varied considerably among all laser-treated eyes of the two treatment groups.

Optic disk photos and retinal sections from the hypertensive (right) eye and normotensive (left) eye of a vehicle-treated animal with very high IOP are shown in Figure 4-4. In the normotensive eye, the perifoveal RGC layer is six or seven cells thick. In the eye with high IOP of 16 months duration, the RGC layer is reduced to a single layer of cells, which are likely predominantly displaced amacrine cells. This hypertensive eye has clearly sustained a severe injury as indicated by an almost complete loss of RGCs. However, this injury is not associated with any obvious change in the morphologic appearance of any other retinal layer. There is no evidence for loss of cells in the outer nuclear layer (photoreceptor cells) or inner nuclear layer (horizontal cells, bipolar cells, Müeller cells, amacrine cells). Of course, subtle changes in cell morphology or cell density would not be readily evident in these histologic sections. This apparently highly selective injury to RGCs was evident in sections obtained from all eight retinal sample regions (central and peripheral) in the hypertensive eyes that showed evidence of RGC loss and supports the notion that, at least in this model for experimental glaucoma, the injury is very specific to RGCs.

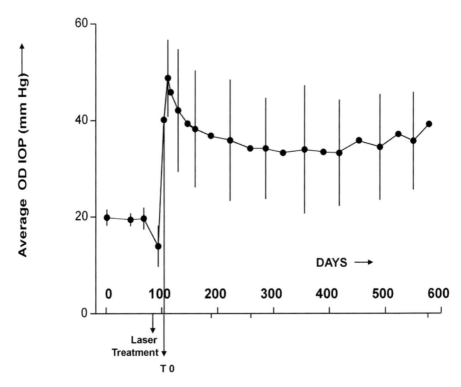

FIGURE 4-3. Mean intraocular pressure (IOP) of all experimental glaucoma eyes in monkey memantine study. Average IOP (± standard deviation) for the hypertensive (OD) eyes of all 18 animals in both treatment groups over the course of the study. (Source: Hare WA, WoldeMussie E, Lai RK, et al. Efficacy and safety of memantine treatment for reduction of changes associated with experimental glaucoma in monkey, I: Functional measures. *Invest Ophthalmol Vis Sci* 2004;45:2625–2639.)

Severe COHT-induced RGC loss was associated with little or no effect on conventional ERG responses to either diffuse flash or 30-Hz flicker stimuli. Because these ERG responses reflect RGC activity to only a small degree, they do not provide a good measure of RGC function. These conventional ERG responses do reflect contributions from activity in most other retinal cell types, and results from these recordings showed that even in animals with severe RGC loss there was little or no effect on the function of other (non-RGC) retinal cells. This functional finding also reinforces the conclusion, based on examination of histologic retinal sections, that COHT injury is very selective for RGCs in this model.

Normotensive (OS)   Hypertensive (OD)

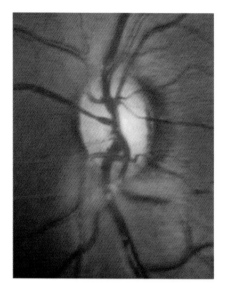
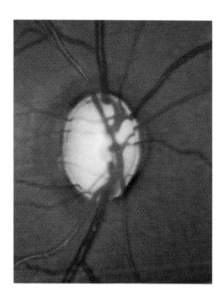

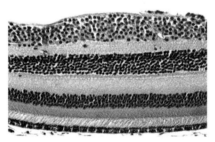
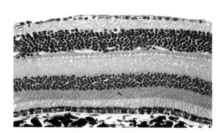

GCL

INL

OPL

ONL

FIGURE 4-4. Experimental glaucoma in a monkey model. Fundus images from the hypertensive right eye and normotensive left eye of a vehicle-treated animal. Micrographs shown directly below the fundus images are hematoxylin-eosin–labeled sections from the perifoveal region (where the RGC density is greatest) obtained from the same eye shown in the fundus image above. (Source: Hare WA, WoldeMussie E, Weinreb RN, et al. Efficacy and safety of memantine treatment for reduction of changes associated with experimental glaucoma in monkey, II: Structural measures. *Invest Ophthalmol Vis Sci* 2004;45:2640–2651.)

Unlike the results with conventional ERG recordings, COHT was associated with a reduction in amplitude of specific multifocal ERG response components. The multifocal ERG provides a spatially discrete map of retinal function over a large retinal area. The multifocal ERG, unlike the conventional ERG responses, also contains components that reflect the activity of RGCs. These same multifocal ERG components had amplitudes that were highly correlated with histologic measures of RGC injury, whereas the other components, in the same manner as the conventional responses, were not affected by COHT injury. The multifocal ERG provides a measure of RGC function/injury. In memantine-treated animals, COHT was associated with less reduction of RGC response components in the multifocal ERG (data not shown). This effect of memantine treatment was seen only at 3 and 5 months after IOP elevation. At the 16-month time point, there were no statistically significant differences between the two treatment groups.

Although ERG measures of RGC function showed a protective effect of memantine treatment at only early time points in the study, RGC counts from sections obtained at 16 months from animals with moderate pressure elevation showed a significant preservation of RGCs in the inferior retina (Fig. 4-5). The Heidelberg Retinal Tomograph measures also showed that memantine treatment was associated with less COHT-induced change in nerve head topography. This treatment effect was seen for measures of both the physiologic cup and neuroretinal rim (data not shown).

VECP recordings obtained at 16 months after IOP elevation provided a rather surprising result. Figure 4-6 shows that hypertensive eyes from three animals in each treatment group had lost most of their RGCs by 16 months. Figure 4-6 also shows that the three eyes from the memantine-treated animals produced VECP responses of normal amplitude, whereas two of the three eyes from vehicle-treated animals had severe attenuation of the VECP response. Because the VECP response reflects activity in visual cortex, it relies completely on the function of RGCs to conduct the visual signal from the retina to more central areas of the CNS. Because RGCs are lost as the result of COHT-induced injury, a given retinal stimulus will drive less cortical response and VECP amplitude will decrease. This is precisely what is seen for the vehicle-treated animals. The fact that severe RGC loss is not

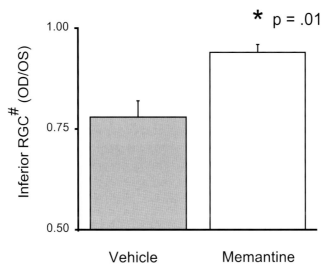

FIGURE 4-5. Memantine treatment was associated with preservation of RGCs in the inferior retina. Summary of normalized (OD/OS) RGC counts from the inferior retina for the four eyes with moderate IOP elevation in each of the two treatment groups. (Source: Hare WA, WoldeMussie E, Weinreb RN, et al. Efficacy and safety of memantine treatment for reduction of changes associated with experimental glaucoma in monkey, II: Structural measures. *Invest Ophthalmol Vis Sci* 2004;45:2640–2651.)

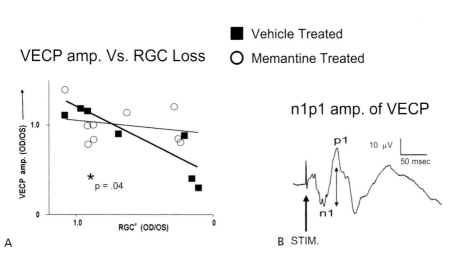

FIGURE 4-6. Visually evoked cortical potential (VECP) responses are well preserved in memantine-treated animals with severe RGC loss. **A:** Plot of peak VECP amplitude, plotted as a function of RGC survival. **B:** Response from stimulation of a normotensive (OS) eye. (Source: Hare WA, WoldeMussie E, Lai RK, et al. Efficacy and safety of memantine treatment for reduction of changes associated with experimental glaucoma in monkey, I: Functional measures. *Invest Ophthalmol Vis Sci* 2004;45:2635.)

associated with decreased VECP amplitude in the memantine-treated animals suggests that memantine treatment may enhance the connections between surviving RGCs and their central targets; that is, memantine treatment may be associated with plastic changes in the synaptic connections at more central levels of the visual pathway. Recently published results from histologic analysis of the lateral geniculate nucleus in memantine-treated monkeys with experimental glaucoma show that memantine treatment is associated with preservation of relay neurons in the lateral geniculate nucleus.[5] This histologic finding is completely consistent with results of functional measures from the present study. This effect of memantine treatment to modify the response of central visual pathways to RGC injury is being examined more closely in ongoing studies.

The normotensive eyes of the two treatment groups of this study provide an opportunity to evaluate whether systemic memantine treatment for 16 months is associated with any effect on normal function of the retina and central visual pathways. The structural and functional measures used to characterize COHT-induced injury were also used to detect any effect of memantine treatment. A comparison of the two treatment groups showed that memantine treatment had no effect on any structural or functional measure in the normotensive eyes (data not shown).

SUMMARY

Results from numerous studies support the notion that overactivity of NMDA-type glutamate channels makes a significant contribution to neuronal injury in a wide range of CNS models, including retina. Results obtained from both rat and monkey models of experimental glaucoma further show that memantine is both safe and effective for the reduction of both structural and functional measures of COHT-induced injury.

REFERENCES

1. WoldeMussie E, Yoles E, Schwartz M, et al. Neuroprotective effect of memantine in different retinal injury models in rats. *J Glaucoma* 2002;11:474–480.

2. Hare WA, WoldeMussie E, Lai RK, et al. Efficacy and safety of memantine treatment for reduction of changes associated with experimental glaucoma in monkey, I: Functional measures. *Invest Ophthalmol Vis Sci* 2004;45:2625–2639.
3. Hare WA, WoldeMussie E, Weinreb RN, et al. Efficacy and safety of memantine treatment for reduction of changes associated with experimental glaucoma in monkey, II: Structural measures. *Invest Ophthalmol Vis Sci* 2004;45:2640–2651.
4. Gaasterland D, Kupfer C. Experimental glaucoma in the rhesus monkey. *Invest Ophthalmol* 1974;13:455–457.
5. Yucel YH, Gupta N, Zhang Q, et al. Memantine protects neurons from shrinkage in the lateral geniculate nucleus in experimental glaucoma. *Arch Ophthalmol* 2005, in press.

5

EVIDENCE FOR NEUROPROTECTION

YENI H. YÜCEL, MD, PHD, FRCPC

The primary injury in glaucoma is at the level of the retinal ganglion cells. However, as in many neurologic diseases, injury can spread to the connected neurons in the brain by a mechanism called "transsynaptic degeneration." In transsynaptic degeneration, target neurons are disconnected from their major afferent pathways, resulting in neuron cell shrinkage and death. Transsynaptic degeneration is a well-known process in Alzheimer's disease, amyotrophic lateral sclerosis, brain trauma, and glaucoma.

GLAUCOMA: A NEURODEGENERATIVE DISEASE OF THE ENTIRE VISUAL SYSTEM

Our laboratory studied the relative changes in different tissue components of the optic nerve and their relationship to nerve fiber loss using an experimental monkey model of glaucoma.[1] In this model, glaucoma was induced in the right eye of eight monkeys using chronic intraocular pressure elevation induced by laser trabeculoplasty. Optic nerve head topographic changes in this model correlated with optic nerve fiber loss. The experimental (right) and control (left) optic nerves were studied using histomorphometric analysis of optic nerve cross sections (Fig. 5-1). The results showed varying degrees of nerve fiber loss in the optic nerves with glaucoma. Glial scar tissue area was significantly increased in optic nerves with severe glaucomatous damage. Although a decrease in total optic nerve area was observed, only myelinated nerve fiber area decreased significantly among the optic nerve tissue components.

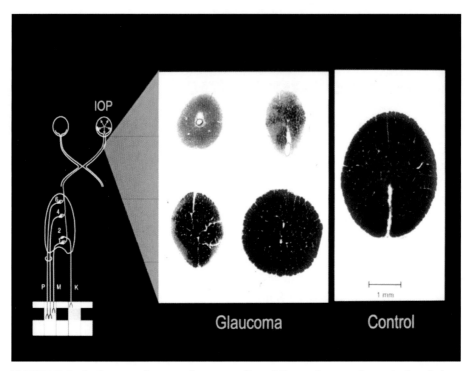

FIGURE 5-1. Optic nerve damage. A cross section of the optic nerve in control and glaucoma. The loss of the black myelin staining indicates optic nerve fiber damage and replacement by glial cells. (Source: Yücel YH, Kalichman MW, Mizisin AP, et al. Histomorphometric analysis of optic nerve changes in experimental glaucoma. *J Glaucoma* 1999;8:38–45.)

The loss of afferent optic nerve fibers in glaucoma is associated with neuronal changes in target central visual neurons. Ninety percent of optic nerve fibers that arise from retinal ganglion cells terminate in a deep structure of the brain called the *lateral geniculate nucleus* (LGN) (Fig. 5-2). Neurons in the LGN convey visual information to the visual cortex.

Understanding neuronal changes in the LGN provides some insight into the affected pathways causing vision loss in glaucoma. Studies in primates have shown that the LGN is organized into at least three distinct LGN neuronal populations occupying separate layers: magnocellular, parvocellular, and koniocellular[2] (Fig. 5-3). Magnocellular neurons convey broadband, luminance contrast,

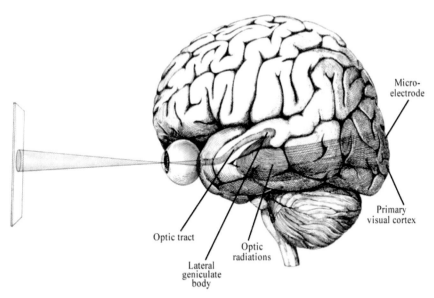

FIGURE 5-2. Visual pathways in the cortex. (Source: Hubel DH. *Eye, Brain, and Vision.* New York: Henry Holt & Co; 1995.)

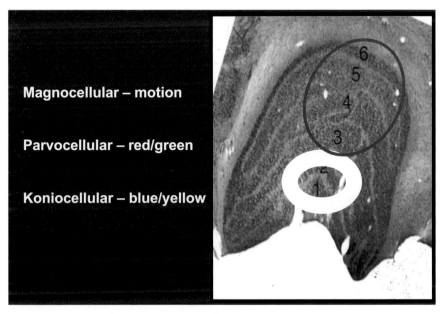

FIGURE 5-3. Lateral geniculate nucleus (LGN). (Source: Yücel YH, Zhang Q, Gupta N, et al. Loss of neurons in magnocellular and parvocellular layers of the lateral geniculate nucleus in glaucoma. *Arch Ophthalmol* 2000;118:378–384.)

and motion signals. Parvocellular neurons convey green-red color opponent signals. Koniocellular neurons, located between the layers, convey blue-on-yellow signals.

In a study of experimental glaucoma in monkeys, there was a significant loss of LGN relay neurons that specifically convey visual information to the primary visual cortex (Fig. 5-4). In this study, four monkeys with experimentally induced glaucoma and five control monkeys were studied. Compared with the control group, the mean number of neurons in the glaucoma group was significantly decreased in magnocellular layer 1 ($P = .02$) and parvocellular layers 4 and 6 ($P = .03$). In glaucomatous LGNs, the cell bodies appeared smaller and fewer in layers 4 and 6 (Fig. 5-5).

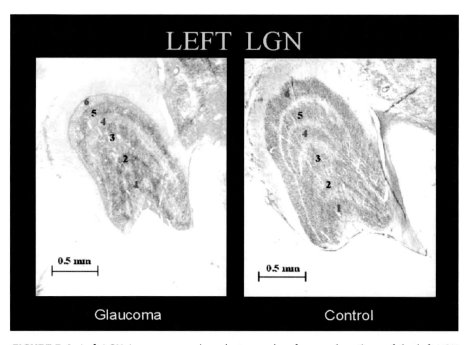

FIGURE 5-4. Left LGN. Low-power microphotographs of coronal sections of the left LGN from control (*right*) and glaucomatous (*left*) monkeys, immunostained for parvalbumin. All six layers in the control are strongly immunoreactive for parvalbumin as indicated by the numbers. There is overall shrinkage of the LGN and a decrease in immunoreactivity in parvocellular layers 4 and 6 in the glaucomatous LGN compared with the control. (Source: Yücel YH, Zhang Q, Gupta N, et al. Loss of neurons in magnocellular and parvocellular layers of the lateral geniculate nucleus in glaucoma. *Arch Ophthalmol* 2000;118:378–384.)

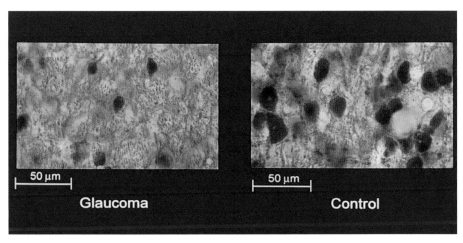

FIGURE 5-5. Relay LGN neurons. High-power micrographs of LGN coronal sections show parvalbumin-immunoreactive neurons in layer 6 of control (*right*) and glaucomatous (*left*) monkeys. In the controls, the darkly stained cell bodies are plump and numerous; in the glaucomatous monkeys, they are shrunken and few. (Source: Yücel YH, Zhang Q, Gupta N, et al. Loss of neurons in magnocellular and parvocellular layers of the lateral geniculate nucleus in glaucoma. *Arch Ophthalmol* 2000;118:378–384.)

Another study using the experimental monkey glaucoma model showed that relay neurons in the LGN undergo significant shrinkage in glaucoma and that neurons in parvocellular layers undergo significantly more shrinkage than neurons in magnocellular layers.[3] In this study, seven monkeys with unilateral experimentally induced glaucoma and five control monkeys were studied.

The results showed an increase in the frequency of the smaller neurons in the glaucoma group compared with the control group, along with a corresponding decrease in the frequency of larger neurons. The mean cross-sectional area of relay neurons in magnocellular layer 1 and parvocellular layers 4 and 6 were significantly decreased in glaucoma compared with controls by 28%, 37%, and 45%, respectively. Neuronal area decreased in a linear fashion for all three layers (Fig. 5-6). The percentage of neuronal shrinkage in each of parvocellular layers 4 and 6, as a function of optic nerve fiber loss, was greater than that seen in magnocellular layer 1 (Fig. 5-7 and Fig 5-8).

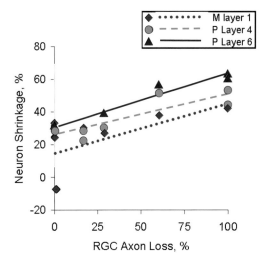

FIGURE 5-6. Neuronal area percentage decrease. Plot of neuronal area percentage decrease for layers 1, 4, and 6 as a function of percentage of retinal ganglion cell loss. (Source: Yücel YH, Zhang Q, Weinreb RN, et al. Atrophy of relay neurons in magno- and parvocellular layers in the lateral geniculate nucleus in experimental glaucoma. *Invest Ophthalmol Vis Sci* 2001;42:3216–3222.)

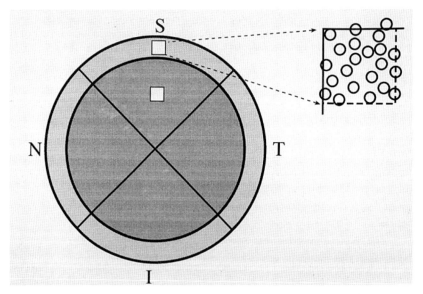

FIGURE 5-7. Optic nerve fiber counts. Each nerve cross section was divided into four quadrants by two meridional lines. Each quadrant was divided into peripheral and central sectors. Two white frames in the superior quadrant indicate the position where six counting frames were placed in the peripheral and central sectors. The insert on the right shows unbiased counting of circles representing optic nerve fibers. Only the profiles completely inside the frame and those intersecting the lower or right-hand border of the frame were counted. The area of each counting frame was 100 μm². S, T, I, and N = superior, temporal, inferior, and nasal quadrants, respectively. (Source: Yücel YH, Gupta N, Kalichman MW, et al. Relationship of optic disc topography to optic nerve fiber number in glaucoma. *Arch Ophthalmol* 1998;116:493–497.)

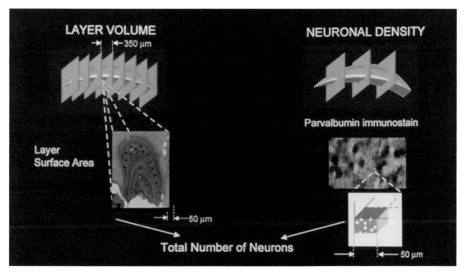

FIGURE 5-8. Three-dimensional morphometry of the magnocellular and parvocellular layers in the LGN. The number of neurons in each layer was calculated by multiplying the average density of neurons (neurons per cubic millimeter) by the layer volume.

NEUROPROTECTION WITH MEMANTINE

The studies described show that in glaucoma, the disease process is not limited to the eye. Glaucoma is a neurodegenerative disease of the entire visual system, including the brain centers. Several mechanisms of neural degeneration have become evident in recent years, including glutamate excitotoxicity, nerve growth factor deprivation, ischemia, autoimmune reactions, and oxidative damage.[4]

Many studies are underway to find medications that protect the optic nerve and retinal ganglion cells. Neuroprotective treatment strategies may stop neural degeneration and promote regeneration in the visual system. Potential strategies under consideration include glutamate N-methyl-D-aspartate (NMDA) receptor blockade, nitric oxide synthase, nerve growth factors, antioxidants, gene therapy, and neural grafts with stem cells.

Memantine is a neuroprotective agent that blocks the NMDA-type glutamatergic excitotoxicity that has been implicated as a mechanism for injury associated with ischemic and other damage to neurons in many regions of the central nervous system. As an NMDA antagonist of the "open channel blocker" type, memantine binds within the channel to a site that is not accessible unless the channel has previously been activated by glutamate binding to a different receptor site. Memantine is both efficacious and well tolerated in the treatment of Parkinson's disease and dementia, and is currently U.S. Food and Drug Administration approved for the treatment of Alzheimer's disease.[5] Clinical trials are currently underway to assess the efficacy of memantine in other neurodegenerative diseases, including glaucoma. In animals, memantine has been shown to reduce retinal injury in experimental glaucoma models, including those induced by ocular hypertension,[6,7] glutamate toxicity,[6,7] ischemia/reperfusion,[8,9] and partial optic nerve crush.[7]

We recently carried out a study to assess the effects of memantine on LGN relay neuron degeneration, using the primate glaucoma model described above.[10] The results of this study were not available (or in press) at the time of publication.

SUMMARY

In experimental primate glaucoma, significant shrinkage and cell death occur in the relay neurons in the LGN, particularly in magnocellular layer 1 and parvocellular layers 4 and 6. Preclinical trials are currently underway to assess the neuroprotective effects of memantine on transsynaptic atrophy of LGN neurons in experimental primate glaucoma.

REFERENCES

1. Yücel YH, Kalichman MW, Mizisin AP, et al. Histomorphometric analysis of optic nerve changes in experimental glaucoma. *J Glaucoma* 1999;8:38–45.
2. Yücel YH, Gupta N, Kalichman MW, et al. Relationship of optic disc topography to optic nerve fiber number in glaucoma. *Arch Ophthalmol* 1998;116:493–497.
3. Yücel YH, Zhang Q, Gupta N, et al. Loss of neurons in magnocellular and parvocellular layers of the lateral geniculate nucleus in glaucoma. *Arch Ophthalmol* 2000; 118:378–384.
4. Yücel YH, Zhang Q, Weinreb RN, et al. Atrophy of relay neurons in magno- and parvocellular layers in the lateral geniculate nucleus in experimental glaucoma. *Invest Ophthalmol Vis Sci* 2001;42:3216–3222.

5. Weinreb RN, Khaw PT. Primary open-angle glaucoma. *Lancet* 2004;363:1711–1720.

6. Reisberg B, Doody R, Stoffler A, et al. Memantine in moderate-to-severe Alzheimer's disease. *N Engl J Med* 2003;348:1333–1341.

7. Gu Z, Yamamoto T, Kawase C, et al. [Neuroprotective effect of N-methyl-D-aspartate receptor antagonists in an experimental glaucoma model in the rat]. *Nippon Ganka Gakkai Zasshi* 2000;104:11–16.

8. WoldeMussie E, Yoles E, Schwartz M, et al. Neuroprotective effect of memantine in different retinal injury models in rats. *J Glaucoma* 2002;11:474–480.

9. Lagreze WA, Knorle R, Bach M, et al. Memantine is neuroprotective in a rat model of pressure-induced retinal ischemia. *Invest Ophthalmol Vis Sci* 1998;39:1063–1066.

10. Osborne NN. Memantine reduces alterations to the mammalian retina, in situ, induced by ischemia. *Vis Neurosci* 1999;16:45–52.

11. Yücel YH, Gupta N, Zhang Q, et al. Memantine protects neurons from shrinkage in the lateral geniculate nucleus in experimental glaucoma. *Arch Ophthalmol* 2006 (in press).

6

ALPHA-2 AGONISTS AND NEURONAL SURVIVAL IN GLAUCOMA

LARRY A. WHEELER, PHD, ELIZABETH WOLDEMUSSIE, PHD, AND RONALD K. LAI, PHD

The alpha-adrenergic system is part of the sympathetic nervous system that controls neuronal excitability. The alpha-adrenergic receptor family consists of two receptor subtypes: the alpha-1 and -2 receptors (Fig. 6-1). In very general terms, activation of the alpha-1 receptors tends to "turn up" the activity of the nervous system, whereas activation of the alpha-2 receptors tends to inhibit neuronal activity.

The alpha-2 adrenergic system can be thought of as one that helps cope with stress. Alpha-2 adrenergic receptors are G_i-coupled receptors that can be activated by endogenous stress hormones such as epinephrine and norepinephrine. Selective alpha-2 agonists activate only the alpha-2 receptors and have minimal or no activity on the alpha-1 receptors. These agonists decrease neuronal excitability and have been shown to be neuroprotective in models of cerebral injury.[1,2]

Alpha-2 receptors are further subdivided into three receptor subtypes: 2A, 2B, and 2C. These receptors can be found in a variety of places in the retina. The alpha-2A gene is expressed in retinal ganglion cells (RGCs) and some cells in the inner nuclear layer (Fig. 6-2). Preliminary data also suggest the presence of alpha-2B and 2C receptors (unpublished data).

When an alpha-2 agonist binds to an alpha-2 adrenergic receptor, a number of signaling mechanisms are initiated by the coupling to G_i proteins (Fig. 6-3). Classically, activation of the alpha-

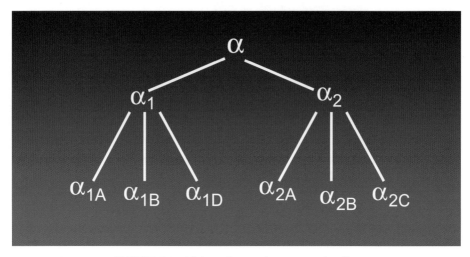

FIGURE 6-1. Alpha adrenergic receptor family.

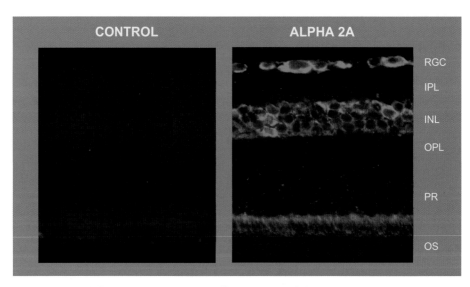

FIGURE 6-2. Alpha-2 receptors are in different parts of the rat retina. Immunolabeling of the retinal with alpha-2A receptor antibody. Alpha-2A receptor is located mainly in the ganglion layer where there are ganglion and amacrine cells. In addition it also stained some amacrine and bipolar cells in the inner nuclear layer.

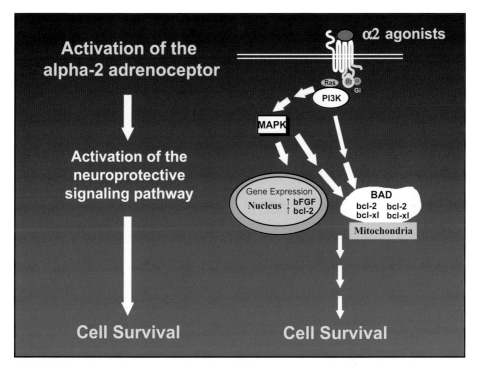

FIGURE 6-3. Alpha-2 receptor activation of the neuroprotective signaling pathway.

2 receptors inhibits adenylyl cyclase, resulting in lowering of intracellular cyclic adenosine monophosphate. In recent years, other second messenger signaling cascades have also been identified. One is the activation of the antiapoptotic phosphatidyl inositol-3 kinase/Akt pathway, which is involved in protecting the mitochondria, key decision makers in cell death.[3] The other area is the mitogen-activated protein kinase pathway, which is important in regulating cell proliferation and apoptosis.

A study by Lai et al. demonstrated that oxidative stress results in the loss of mitochondrial membrane potential, and that brimonidine treatment significantly protected the cells expressing alpha-2 receptors (but did not protect the cells not expressing alpha-2 receptors) by helping the mitochondria withstand oxidative stress (unpublished data).

Survival pathways activated by brimonidine are summarized in Figure 6-4. Basically, alpha-2 agonists can activate similar sur-

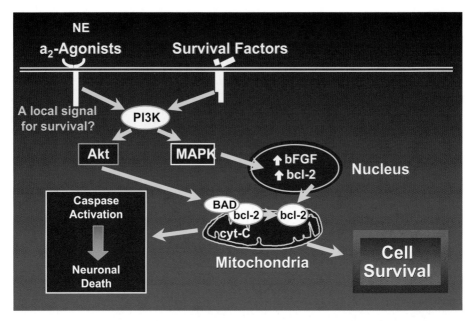

FIGURE 6-4. Survival pathways activated by brimonidine. Activation of the alpha-2 receptors by brimonidine activates phosphatidyl inositol-3 kinase, which subsequently activates Akt (protein kinase B). These are major pathways in the promotion of cell survival.

vival signaling cascades that are activated by other known growth factors such as insulin, basic fibroblast growth factor, and brain-derived neurotrophic factor. Activation of alpha-2 receptors is believed to play a role as a local signal for releasing survival factors, such as B-cell lymphoma-2 (Bcl-2) and B-cell lymphoma-xl (Bcl-xl). The mechanisms by which stimulation of the alpha-2 receptors protect the RGCs are not completely understood. However, activation of survival pathways by alpha-2 agonists may provide local protection when delivery of growth factors or survival factors from the brain is hampered by high intraocular pressure (IOP).

BRIMONIDINE AND NEUROPROTECTION

Brimonidine is a selective alpha-2 adrenergic agonist that is currently used topically to decrease IOP in patients with glaucoma. Brimonidine has been tested in a wide range of model systems, including optic nerve crush,[4] ocular hypertension in the rat,[5–7] pressure-induced ischemia,[8,9] vascular ischemia,[10,11] transgenic mouse-

SOD-1 overexpression,[12] light-induced photoreceptor damage,[13,14] and photoreceptor degeneration.[15] The mechanisms described above are believed to be the basis for its activity in these models.

The neuroprotective effects of brimonidine were assessed in a rat model of chronic ocular hypertension (COHT).[6] In this model, IOP was elevated using laser photocoagulation of the episcleral and limbal veins. Brimonidine or timolol was administered, either at the time of or 10 days after IOP elevation, and continued for 3 weeks. RGC loss was then evaluated in whole mounted retinas.

After 3 weeks of elevated IOP, RGC loss was approximately 35% that of the control. Although systemic application of brimonidine or timolol had little effect on IOP, brimonidine, but not timolol, showed significant protection of RGCs when applied at the time of IOP elevation. Brimonidine treatment reduced the rate of loss by approximately 50% (Fig. 6-5), indicating that neuroprotective activity was unrelated to its effects on ocular hypotension.

The effects of brimonidine on immunoreactivity of intermediate filament glial fibrillary acidic protein (GFAP) were also assessed in a similar experiment. (GFAP is a marker of stress that is classi-

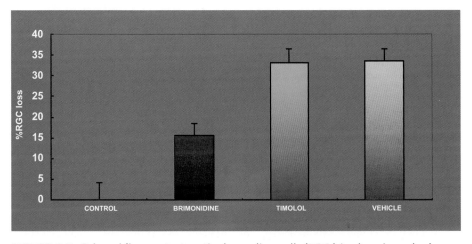

FIGURE 6-5. Brimonidine protects retinal ganglion cells (RGCs) in chronic ocular hypertensive rats. Brimonidine applied at the time of laser treatment and continued for 3 weeks caused 50% prevention of ganglion cell loss. There was a 35% ganglion cell loss in vehicle-treated group. Timolol showed no protective effect.

cally studied in the central nervous system and the retina.) In retinas with normal IOP, GFAP is expressed in the fiber layer only (astrocytes and Müller cell endfeet). After elevation of IOP, GFAP immunoreactivity increased in the Müller cells (Fig. 6-6). Treatment with brimonidine caused a significant decrease in GFAP expression compared with vehicle-treated eyes, whereas treatment with timolol showed no decrease in immunoreactivity of GFAP.

In a different study, the effect of brimonidine initiated after IOP elevation was evaluated. In this study when the animals were exposed to elevated pressure for 10 days, ganglion cell loss was approximately 22% that of control. Brimonidine administration initiated 10 days after IOP elevation prevented any further loss of ganglion cells. In vehicle- or timolol-treated rats, ganglion cell loss continued to 33%[6] (Fig. 6-7).

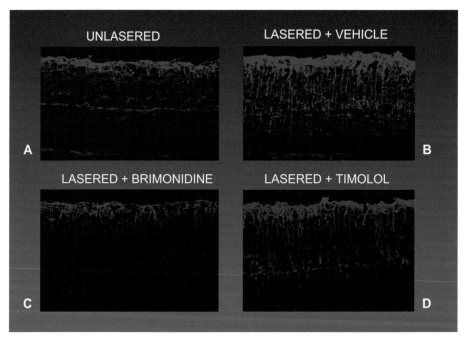

FIGURE 6-6. Glial fibrillary acidic protein (GFAP) immunoreactivity. Immunohistochemical staining of retinas for GFAP. Drugs were administered at the time of IOP elevation. Three weeks later, eyes were fixed and cross-sectioned retinas were stained with anti-GFAP antibody. **A:** GFAP immunostaining in retinas with normal IOP. **B:** Elevation of IOP increased GFAP staining. **C:** Brimonidine caused a significant decrease in GFAP staining (*P = .025). **D:** Timolol caused a slight, nonsignificant decrease.

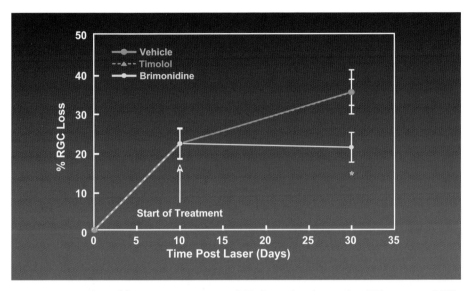

FIGURE 6-7. Brimonidine treatment started 10 days after increasing IOP protects RGCs. Brimonidine-induced neuroprotection of ganglion cells. Brimonidine at 1 mg/kg/day or timolol at 2 mg/kg/day was applied 10 days (*arrow*) after the first laser treatment. There was a 22% decrease in ganglion cells after 10 days. Treatment with brimonidine prevented any further loss of ganglion cells (*P = .05). Timolol had no effect on ganglion cell loss. Values represent mean ± standard error of mean of measurements in 15 rats.

A study by Aviles-Trigueros et al.[10] indicated that brimonidine protected against ischemia-induced degeneration of the retinotectal projection, and preserved anterograde axonal transport. This experiment involved injection of cholera toxin subunit-B (CTB) into the vitreous, based on the theory that if the motor machinery that transports proteins is intact and not injured by stress, the CTB will be transported to the brain. The transport of CTB was assessed by obtaining serial coronal sections of the mesencephalon and brain stem and measuring immunoreactivity for CTB (Fig. 6-8). Areas devoid of CTB immunoreactivity suggest orthograde degeneration of retinal terminals and/or decrease of anterograde axonal transport.[10]

This technique was used in a recent study to compare the neuroprotective effects of topically applied brimonidine-purite (Alphagan® P [Allergan Inc., Irvine, CA] brimonidine tartrate ophthalmic solution 0.15%), timolol, and saline in a rat model of COHT (data not shown).[16] Serial coronal sections of the midbrain were inmunostained for CTB, and the visual layers of the contralateral superior colliculus were examined to estimate the volume of the retinotectal projection. The results showed that treatment with brimonidine provided statistically significant protection against COHT-induced degeneration of the retinotectal projection in this rat model. Timolol treatment did not prevent retinotectal degeneration.

These laboratory findings led to a number of translational clinical research studies. A study by Kent et al.[17] was carried out to determine the vitreous concentration of brimonidine after topical administration in patients undergoing elective pars plana vitrectomy. In this prospective observational case series, brimonidine tartrate 0.2% was topically administered two or three times daily for 4 to 14 days preoperatively in 13 patients. Four patients served as controls,

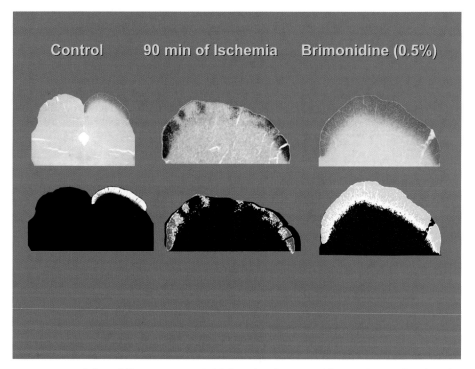

FIGURE 6-8. Brimonidine preserves RGC function in rats with transient ischemia. The transport of CTB can be assessed by obtaining serial sections of the superior colliculus and measuring immunoreactivity for CTB. **A:** Normal unlesioned eye. **B:** Lesioned vehicle treated eye. **C,D:** Lesioned and brimonidine-treated eye. (Source: Aviles-Trigueros M, Mayor-Torroglosa S, Garcia-Aviles A, et al. Transient ischemia of the retina results in massive degeneration of the retinotectal projection: long-term neuroprotection with brimonidine. *Exp Neurol* 2003;184:767–777.)

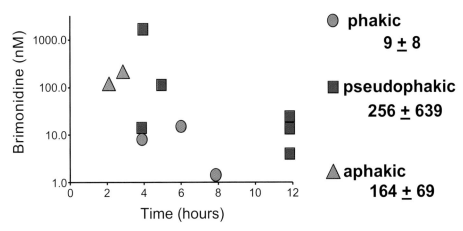

FIGURE 6-9. Human vitreous concentrations of brimonidine: translational clinical research. Vitreal concentration of brimonidine after topical application ranged from 9 to 256 nM. This was higher than the concentration required to stimulate the alpha-2 receptors. (Source: Kent AR, Nussdorf JD, David R, et al. Vitreous concentration of topically applied brimonidine tartrate 0.2%. *Ophthalmology* 2001;108:784–787.)

without application of brimonidine. All patients treated with brimonidine measured above the lower limit of quantitation with a mean vitreous concentration of 185 ± 500 nM. All patients not treated with brimonidine measured at or below the lower limit of quantitation of 0.05 nM. There was a trend toward higher concentration in patients who were either aphakic or pseudophakic compared with those who were phakic (Fig. 6-9). These data suggest that topically applied brimonidine results in vitreous levels at or above the 2 nM concentration that is known to activate alpha-2 receptors.

More recently, Bartholomew et al.[18] carried out a similar study using topically applied brimonidine-purite. As in the previous study, the application of topical brimonidine purite 0.15%, two or three times daily, resulted in vitreous concentrations at or above the concentration required to activate the alpha-2 receptor.

SUMMARY

The alpha-2 adrenoreceptor system also functions to help the retina deal with stress. Activation of the alpha-2 adrenoreceptor pathway with brimonidine protects against optic nerve and retinal injury and cell death.

REFERENCES

1. Reis DJ, Regunathan S, Meeley MP. Imidazole receptors and clonidine-displacing substance in relationship to control of blood pressure, neuroprotection, and adrenomedullary secretion. *Am J Hypertens* 1992;5:51S–57S.
2. Maier C, Steinberg GK, Sun GH, et al. Neuroprotection by the alpha 2-adrenoreceptor agonist dexmedetomidine in a focal model of cerebral ischemia. *Anesthesiology* 1993; 79:306–312.
3. Hunot S, Flavell RA. Apoptosis. Death of a monopoly? *Science* 2001;292:865–866.
4. Yoles E, Wheeler LA, Schwartz M. Alpha2-adrenoreceptor agonists are neuroprotective in a rat model of optic nerve degeneration. *Invest Ophthalmol Vis Sci* 1999;40:65–73.
5. Ahmed FA, Hegazy K, Chaudhary P, et al. Neuroprotective effect of alpha(2) agonist (brimonidine) on adult rat retinal ganglion cells after increased intraocular pressure. *Brain Res* 2001;913:133–139.
6. WoldeMussie E, Ruiz G, Wijono M, et al. Neuroprotection of retinal ganglion cells by brimonidine in rats with laser-induced chronic ocular hypertension. *Invest Ophthalmol Vis Sci* 2001;42:2849–2855.
7. Levkovitch-Verbin H, Harris-Cerruti C, Groner Y, et al. RGC death in mice after optic nerve crush injury: oxidative stress and neuroprotection. *Invest Ophthalmol Vis Sci* 2000;41(13):4169–4181.
8. Lai RK, Chun T, Hasson D, et al. Alpha-2 adrenoceptor agonist protects retinal function after acute retinal ischemic injury in the rat. *Vis Neurosci* 2002;19:175–185.
9. Donello JE, Padillo EU, Webster ML, et al. alpha(2)-Adrenoceptor agonists inhibit vitreal glutamate and aspartate accumulation and preserve retinal function after transient ischemia. *J Pharmacol Exp Ther* 2001;296:216–223.
10. Aviles-Trigueros M, Mayor-Torroglosa S, Garcia-Aviles A, et al. Transient ischemia of the retina results in massive degeneration of the retinotectal projection: long-term neuroprotection with brimonidine. *Exp Neurol* 2003;184:767–777.
11. Lafuente MP, Villegas-Perez MP, Mayor S, et al. Neuroprotective effects of brimonidine against transient ischemia-induced retinal ganglion cell death: a dose response in vivo study. *Exp Eye Res* 2002;74:181–189.

12. Schori H, Kipnis J, Yoles E, et al. Vaccination for protection of retinal ganglion cells against death from glutamate cytotoxicity and ocular hypertension: implications for glaucoma. *Proc Natl Acad Sci U S A* 2001;98(6):3398–3403. Epub 2001

13. Wen R, Cheng T, Li Y, et al. Alpha 2-adrenergic agonists induce basic fibroblast growth factor expression in photoreceptors in vivo and ameliorate light damage. *J Neurosci* 1996;16(19):5986–5992.

14. Lai R, Chun T. Effect of A$_2$ adrenoceptor agonist, brimonidine, in a blue light-induced retinal degeneration model. *Invest Ophthalmol Vis Sci* 2001;42:S629 (abstract).

15. Ervin CS, Wohabrebbi A, Innaccone M, et al. Brimonidine rescues photoreceptors from degeneration induced by retinal pigment epithelium removal in vitro. *Invest Ophthalmol Vis Sci* 1999;40:858 (abstract).

16. Mayor-Torroglosa S, WoldeMussie E, Ruiz G, et al. Laser-induced chronic ocular hypertension results in degeneration of retino-tectal afferents: neuroprotection with topical brimonidine. *Invest Ophthalmol Vis Sci* 2004;45:877 (abstract).

17. Kent AR, Nussdorf JD, David R, et al. Vitreous concentration of topically applied brimonidine tartrate 0.2%. *Ophthalmology* 2001;108:784–787.

18. Bartholomew LR, Kent AR, King L. Vitreous concentration of topically applied brimonidine-purite 0.15%. *Invest Ophthalmol Vis Sci* 2005;46:1325 (abstract).

7

NEURONAL DEGENERATION: PROTECTION WITH ALPHA-2 AGONISTS

MANUEL VIDAL-SANZ, MD, PHD

Over the last few years, our laboratory has studied several models to assess the effects of retinal injury-induced neuronal cell death. We have examined the effects of axotomy-induced retinal injury, transient ischemia-induced retinal injury, and ocular hypertension-induced retinal injury. At the same time, we have also been exploring the possibility of halting or preventing the effects of the injury-induced cell degeneration through neuroprotection.

This chapter reviews our laboratory's work on the effects of transient ischemia of the retina induced by selective ligature of the ophthalmic vessels (LOVs) and the protective effects of brimonidine (BMD) against this injury. We assessed the effects of LOV-induced transient ischemia on retinal ganglion cells (RCGs) using a rat model[1] and found that the severity and duration of loss of the RGCs were related to the length of the ischemic interval. For instance, after 90 minutes of transient ischemia of the retina, approximately 40% of the RGC population was lost by 5 days, and RGC loss continued for an additional 2 to 3 months[2] (Fig. 7-1).

Subsequent studies were carried out to determine whether this dramatic RGC loss could be prevented by applying molecules with neuroprotective properties.[1,3] The remainder of this discussion will focus on our work with BMD, an alpha-2 selective agonist.[4]

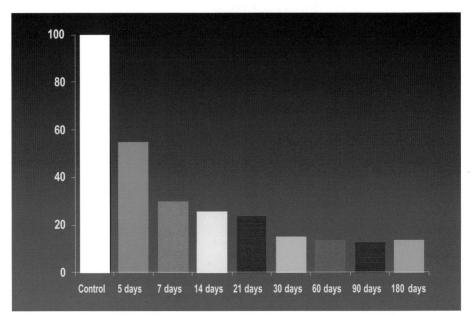

FIGURE 7-1. Retinal ganglion cell (RGC) survival after 90 minutes of ligature of the ophthalmic vessels (LOV): Percentage of di-ASP-labeled RGCs. Transient LOV for 90 minutes results in progressive RGC loss. Data represent mean densities (expressed as percentages of control retinas) of di-ASP-labeled RGCs in the left experimental retinas of groups of rats at increasing survival periods of time (5–180 days) after 90 minutes LOV. RGC death begins during the first 5 days and progresses for up to 2 months. (Source: Lafuente MP, Villegas-Perez MP, Selles-Navarro I, et al. Retinal ganglion cell death after acute retinal ischemia is an ongoing process whose severity and duration depends on the duration of the insult. *Neuroscience* 2002;109:157–168.)

NEUROPROTECTIVE EFFECTS OF BRIMONIDINE AGAINST ISCHEMIA-INDUCED RETINAL CELL DEATH

In recent studies, we found that a single instillation of two drops of 0.5% BMD into the left eye resulted in a significant activation of survival factors and in the upregulation of the expression of trophic factors in that retina.[5] When applied topically to the left eye of rats, BMD was found to be neuroprotective against retinal ischemia in a dose-dependent manner.[6] The 0.1% concentration achieved optimal neuroprotective effects against the early loss of RGCs, and maximum effects were achieved with 0.5%. Neuroprotection lasted for up to 21 days after the injury and was also observed when BMD was administered 1 or 2 hours after the injury.[7]

A number of studies were then carried out to examine the effects of retinal ischemia on the inner retinal layers and the rest of the brain. The full-field electroretinogram recording technique was used to assess inner and outer retinal layer function after ischemia-induced retinal damage. Three months after ischemia, the b-wave amplitudes in the vehicle-treated eyes were significantly smaller when compared with the contralateral normal eye. The BMD-treated group showed no significant differences between the injured eye and the normal eye.[8]

The retinas were also assessed morphologically in cross sections. In the vehicle-treated group, the thickness of the inner nuclear layer and the inner plexiform layer had decreased by approximately one-third, whereas in the BMD-treated group, there was no significant loss.[8]

Another study documented that not all of the RGCs that survived ischemia retained their capacity for retrograde axonal transport.[9] In addition, the results showed that in BMD-pretreated animals, the densities of tracer-labeled RGCs were similar to those found in their contralateral eyes (Fig. 7-2). These findings suggested that the RGCs that were rescued from ischemia-induced cell death with BMD retained their physiologic capacity for retrograde and orthograde axonal transport[9,10] (Fig. 7-3).

EFFECTS OF ISCHEMIA AFTER THREE MONTHS: NEUROPROTECTION WITH BRIMONIDINE

In a recent study,[8] the effects of ischemia on the inner and outer retina and on the retinofugal projection were examined 3 months after transient ischemia of the retina in a rat model. Neuroprotective effects of BMD were also assessed. In this model, the left eye of adult rats was subjected to 90 minutes of LOV. One hour before ischemia, two drops of saline alone or saline containing 0.5% BMD were instilled in the eye. The retinotectal projection was orthograde-labeled with cholera toxin subunit B (CTB), injected in the eye, and measured in serial coronal sections of the superior colliculus.

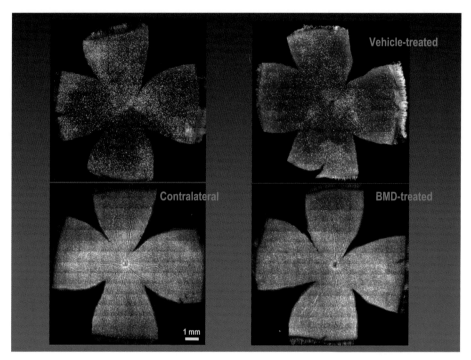

FIGURE 7-2. Retinal ischemia alters retrograde axoplasmic transport: Neuroprotection with brimonidine (BMD). Photographic reconstructions of two representative whole-mounted left retinas in experimental rats pretreated with topical saline in the left eye (top retinas, vehicle-treated) or with 0.5% BMD (BMD-treated), 1 hour before 90 minutes of transient ischemia of the left eye. RGCs that would preserve their retrograde axonal transport were identified with the tracer FluoroGold (FG) applied to both superior colliculi 7 days after ischemia. Rats were processed 1 week later. In the vehicle-treated retinas, FG-labeled RGCs appear scattered with focal areas lacking RGCs, whereas in the BMD-treated retina, FG-labeled RGCs appeared evenly distributed throughout the retinal quadrants in both the ischemic (BMD-treated) and fellow nonischemic (contralateral) retina. The superior aspect of the retinas is between the 1- and 2-o'clock orientations. (Source: Lafuente Lopez-Herrera MP, Mayor-Torroglosa S, Miralles de Imperial J, et al. Transient ischemia of the retina results in altered retrograde axoplasmic transport: neuroprotection with brimonidine. *Exp Neurol* 2002;178:243–258.)

In the unlesioned (control) rat, very densely CTB-labeled retinal axons filled the superficial layers of the superior colliculus. In contrast, CTB-labeled profiles were reduced in the vehicle-treated rat. In the BMD group, the densities of CTB-labeled profiles were significantly greater than those in the vehicle-treated group, indicating a prevention of the ischemia-induced effect on projection.

Vehicle-treated

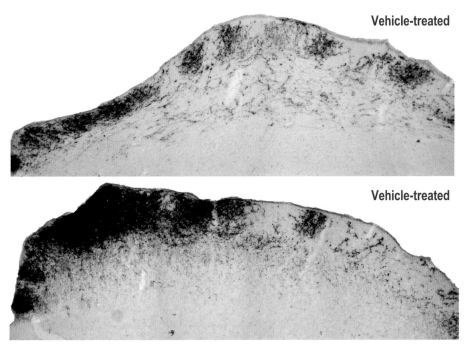

Vehicle-treated

FIGURE 7-3. Retinal ischemia results in massive degeneration of retinotectal terminals. In coronal sections of the midbrain, light micrographs show the distribution of retinal afferents to the visual layers of the superior colliculus in two rats, 2 months after 90 minutes of retinal ischemia. Retinal axons were identified with the orthograde tracer cholera toxin subunit B (CTB) injected intraocularly 5 days before sacrifice and serial sectioning of the midbrain. In contrast with unlesioned control animals, the vehicle-treated animals show marked reductions of CTB-labeled profiles, with areas that were virtually lacking CTB-immunoreactive fibers. (Source: Aviles-Trigueros M, Mayor-Torroglosa S, Garcia-Aviles A, et al. Transient ischemia of the retina results in massive degeneration of the retinotectal projection: long-term neuroprotection with brimonidine. *Exp Neurol* 2003;184:767–777.)

The CTB-labeled profiles were quantified for each animal by using computerized image and mathematic analysis. The volume of the retinofugal projection to the contralateral superior colliculus was estimated as an indication of the integrity of the major retinal output to the brain. The results indicated that approximately one-third of the entire retinotectal projection volume was lost 3 months after 90 minutes of retinal ischemia. BMD administration significantly protected against this retinal damage and degeneration of retinal projection.[8]

SUMMARY

After 3 months, retinal ischemia induces profound functional and structural alterations of the inner and RGC layers, and of the main retinofugal projection. These findings reflect the degeneration of the inner retinal layers, the RGC population, and the retinotectal projection. Functionally, this implies a permanent disconnection of the retina from its main retinorecipient target region in the brain. Alpha-2 selective agonists such as BMD may prevent or diminish ischemia-induced alterations of the inner and RGC layers and at the main retinofugal projection.

REFERENCES

1. Vidal-Sanz M, Lafuente MP, Selles-Navarro I, et al. Retinal ischemia. In: Levin LA, DiPolo A, eds. *Ocular neuroprotection.* New York: Marcel Dekker Inc; 2003:129–152.
2. Lafuente MP, Villegas-Perez MP, Selles-Navarro I, et al. Retinal ganglion cell death after acute retinal ischemia is an ongoing process whose severity and duration depends on the duration of the insult. *Neuroscience* 2002;109:157–168.
3. Vidal-Sanz M, Lafuente MP, Sobrado-Calvo P, et al. Neuroprotection of retinal ganglion cells after different types of injury. *Neurotoxicity Res* 2000;2:215–227.
4. Vidal-Sanz M, Lafuente MP, Mayor-Torroglosa S, et al. Brimonidine's neuroprotective effects against transient ischaemia-induced retinal ganglion cell death. *Eur J Ophthalmol* 2001;11 (Suppl 2):S36–S40.
5. Napankangas U, Lafuente MP, Lindqvist N, et al. Expression of the pro-apoptotic BH3-only protein beam after optic nerve axotomy and transient retinal ischemia. *Invest Ophthalmol Vis Sci* 2004;45:(E-Abstract)3264.
6. Lafuente MP, Villegas-Perez MP, Mayor S, et al. Neuroprotective effects of brimonidine against transient ischemia-induced retinal ganglion cell death: a dose response in vivo study. *Exp Eye Res* 2002;74:181–189.
7. Lafuente MP, Villegas-Perez MP, Sobrado-Calvo P, et al. Neuroprotective effects of alpha(2)-selective adrenergic agonists against ischemia-induced retinal ganglion cell death. *Invest Ophthalmol Vis Sci* 2001;42:2074–2084.

8. Mayor-Torroglosa S, De la villa P, Rodriguez ME, et al. Ischemia results 3 months later in an altered ERG, degeneration of inner retinal layers, and a deafferented tectum: neuroprotection with brimonidine. *Invest Ophthalmol Vis Sci* 2005;46:3825–3835.

9. Lafuente Lopez-Herrera MP, Mayor-Torroglosa S, Miralles de Imperial J, et al. Transient ischemia of the retina results in altered retrograde axoplasmic transport: neuroprotection with brimonidine. *Exp Neurol* 2002;178:243–258.

10. Aviles-Trigueros M, Mayor-Torroglosa S, Garcia-Aviles A, et al. Transient ischemia of the retina results in massive degeneration of the retinotectal projection: long-term neuroprotection with brimonidine. *Exp Neurol* 2003;184:767–777.

8

MEASURING NEUROPROTECTION IN GLAUCOMA CLINICAL TRIALS

DAVID S. GREENFIELD, MD

The ability to measure human neuroprotection is fundamentally linked to the clinical measurement of glaucoma progression. Yet, identification of surrogate markers for glaucoma progression remains a challenge for clinicians and investigators. An ideal progression monitor would be highly sensitive, specific, and resistant to fluctuation. Such a monitor would require very few confirmatory tests and have broad sensitivity ranges throughout the entire glaucoma continuum. To be widely used, such a monitor should also be easy to interpret. Most currently available ancillary tests for glaucoma diagnosis and monitoring do not satisfy all of these characteristics.

At the present time, standard efficacy end points in human glaucoma clinical trials include reproducible change in visual function using standard automated perimetry (SAP), and change in optic disc appearance using stereoscopic optic disc photography. Although such end points have been well validated, considerable limitations exist. Glaucoma progression occurs slowly, and changes are often subtle and easily missed. Many confirmatory visual fields are often required to differentiate test–retest variability from physiologic change. In the Ocular Hypertension Treatment Study, suspected visual field progression was not confirmed in 86% of eyes with repeat testing.[1] In the collaborative normal-tension glaucoma study, 57% of eyes with suspected progression were false positives.[2] These studies suggested that perhaps as much as four confirmatory visual fields may be required to substantiate suspected visual field progression. Randomized clinical trials in glaucoma are therefore costly and of long duration.

MEASURING PROGRESSION IN CLINICAL TRIALS

Glaucoma progression in clinical trials is often characterized using predefined end points. This is a strategy known as event-based progression. Although this strategy provides a standardized approach, there has been poor consensus among randomized clinical trials regarding the definition of a visual field end point. Rate-based progression represents an alternative approach that describes glaucoma progression as a function of parameter-based change over time. Rate-based progression strategies have not been widely adopted in clinical trials.

Table 8-1 summarizes some of the criteria for visual field progression in glaucoma randomized clinical trials. A limitation of event-based progression strategies is that most patients never reach an efficacy end point, resulting in underuse of clinical data. Furthermore, functional end points such as visual fields have considerable variability resulting in the need for multiple confirmatory tests to increase specificity. Table 8-2 describes the efficacy end points achieved in four glaucoma clinical trials in which a treated

TABLE 8-1. SUMMARIZED DEFINITIONS OF VISUAL FIELD PROGRESSION IN GLAUCOMA RANDOMIZED CLINICAL TRIALS

Ocular Hypertension Treatment Study (OHTS)[3]	3 points on pattern deviation plot ($P \leq 5\%$) on 3 consecutive visual fields
Advanced Glaucoma Intervention Study (AGIS)[26]	Increase in baseline score ≥ 4 on 3 consecutive visual fields
Collaborative Initial Glaucoma Treatment Study (CIGTS)[27]	Increase in baseline score ≥ 3 on 3 consecutive visual fields
Early Manifest Glaucoma Trial (EMGT)[5]	≥ 3 points worse on 3 consecutive glaucoma change probability maps
Normal Tension Glaucoma Study (NTGS)[6,7]	≥ 2 points decreased ≥ 10 dB on 4 consecutive visual fields
Glaucoma Laser Trial (GLT)[28]	≥ 1 point decreased ≥ 7–11 dB on 3 consecutive visual fields
Fluorouracil Filtering Surgery Study (FFSS)[29]	Not defined (not an outcome variable)

TABLE 8-2. NUMBER OF PATIENTS ACHIEVING STANDARD EFFICACY END POINTS IN GLAUCOMA CLINICAL TRIALS WITH TREATMENT AND OBSERVATIONAL COHORTS

Clinical Trial	Treated		Observation	
	VF	Disc	VF	Disc
Ocular Hypertension Treatment Study (OHTS)[3]	15	18	29	51
European Glaucoma Prevention Study (EGPS)[4]	26	21	38	22
Early Manifest Glaucoma Trial (EMGT)[5]	53	1	64	0
Collaborative Normal-tension Glaucoma Study Group (CNTGS)[6,7]	6	1	25	3

cohort was compared with an observational control population. The Ocular Hypertension Treatment Study[3] and European Glaucoma Prevention Study[4] involved subjects with elevated intraocular pressure but normal standard fields and optic discs at entry. Standard efficacy end points were achieved in only 8% to 10% of patients. In eyes further along in the glaucoma continuum, such as those eyes in the Early Manifest Glaucoma Trial[5] or in the Collaborative Normal-tension Glaucoma Study,[6,7] efficacy end points were seen in 25% to 50% of patients.

There are presently three human clinical neuroprotection trials (Table 8-3). One study seeks to evaluate the effectiveness and safety of oral memantine, a noncompetitive N-methyl-D-aspartate antagonist, in patients with chronic open-angle glaucoma who are at risk for progression of the disease. The primary end point is a change in SAP, and secondary end points include optic disc photography and frequency doubling technology (FDT). The Low-pressure Glaucoma Treatment Study[8] is investigating visual field stability in patients with low-pressure glaucoma randomized to in-

TABLE 8-3. CURRENT HUMAN GLAUCOMA NEUROPROTECTION TRIALS

Clinical Trial	Primary End Point	Secondary End Points
Memantine	SAP	ODP, FDT
Low-pressure Glaucoma Treatment Study (LoGTS)[8]	SAP	ODP
Brimonidine vs. ALT	SAP	

ALT, argon laser trabeculoplasty; SAP, standard automated perimetry; ODP, optic disc photography; FDT, frequency doubling technology.

traocular pressure reduction in both eyes with topical twice-daily brimonidine tartrate 0.2% versus twice-daily timolol maleate 0.5%. Another study is evaluating visual field stability in patients with glaucoma who are randomized to receive brimonidine 0.2% versus argon laser trabeculoplasty. In both of these studies, the primary end point is SAP.

FUNCTIONAL AND STRUCTURAL TECHNOLOGIES

A number of technologies (Table 8-4) exist that provide assessment of visual function in patients with glaucoma. SAP (Carl Zeiss Meditec, Dublin, CA) uses a white target presented on a white background and measures retinal threshold sensitivity using a statistical approach that combines staircase target presentations with maximum likelihood assessment. Short-wavelength automated perimetry (SWAP, Carl Zeiss Meditec) uses a blue target presented on a yellow background and measures koniocellular retinal ganglion cell function. SWAP may detect glaucomatous visual field loss up to 5 years before SAP. FDT (Carl Zeiss Meditec) uses a sinusoidal grating with low spatial frequency and a rapid counterphase that measures magnocellular retinal ganglion cell function. There is evidence that FDT[9] and SWAP[10] abnormalities precede SAP visual field loss by as much as 4 and 5 years, respectively, in ocular hypertensive eyes and patients with suspected glaucoma. Multifocal visual evoked potential testing[11]

TABLE 8-4. TECHNOLOGIES FOR ASSESSMENT OF VISUAL FUNCTION

Technology	Principle	Normative Data	Primary Function
SAP	White on white	Yes	Nonselective RGC function
SWAP	Blue on yellow	Yes	Koniocellular RGC function
FDT	Motion sensitive	Yes	Magnocellular RGC function
PERG	ERG	Yes	Nonselective RGC function
MVEP	VEP	No	Parvocellular and magnocellular RGC function

SAP, standard automated perimetry; SWAP, short-wavelength automated perimetry; FDT, frequency doubling technology; PERG, pattern electroretinogram; MVEP, multifocal visual evoked potential; RGC, retinal ganglion cell.

TABLE 8-5. TECHNOLOGIES FOR ASSESSMENT OF GLAUCOMATOUS STRUCTURAL DAMAGE

Technology	Principle	Normative Data	Primary Function
RNFL photograph	Red free light	None	Nonquantitative RNFL assessment
Optic disc photograph	White light	None	Nonquantitative disc assessment
GDx-VCC	Retardation	>500	RNFL assessment
OCT	Interferometry	300	RNFL assessment
HRT	CSLO	<150	Disc topography

RNFL, retinal nerve fiber layer; GDx-VCC, GDx with variable corneal compensation; OCT, optical coherence tomography; HRT, Heidelberg Retinal Tomograph; CSLO, confocal scanning laser tomography.

and the pattern electroretinogram[12] (Lace Electronics, Pisa, Italy) represent new strategies that measure electrical signals generated by retinal ganglion cells and provide an objective measure of retinal ganglion cell function.

Various structural technologies exist that have the potential to provide relevant neuroprotective efficacy end points (Table 8-5). Although widely recognized as the standard end point for glaucomatous structural damage, stereoscopic optic disc photography provides nonquantitative information about the optic nerve, and detection of progression is subtle and entirely subjective. The Heidelberg Retinal Tomograph (Heidelberg Engineering, Heidelberg, Germany), is a confocal scanning laser ophthalmoscope that obtains cross-sectional images of the optic nerve and generates a topographic map. It has been studied in the European Glaucoma Prevention Study[4] and in an ancillary study of the Ocular Hypertension Treatment Study,[13] and was recently demonstrated to predict conversion to primary open-angle glaucoma with a predictive power of up to 40%.[13] The Confocal Scanning Laser Tomography Ancillary Study[13] provides the first evidence-based documentation that an imaging technology is valid. The study demonstrates that even when the optic disc is not classified as glaucomatous and the standard visual field is normal, certain optic disc features obtained with confocal scanning laser tomography are significantly associated with the development of glaucoma.

Documentation of retinal nerve fiber layer (RNFL) atrophy in glaucomatous eyes was originally described using red-free

TABLE 8-6. EVIDENCE SUPPORTING DETECTION OF GLAUCOMA PROGRESSION WITH POSTERIOR SEGMENT IMAGING TECHNOLOGIES

Author (Year)	Technology	Sample Size	Diagnosis
Kamal et al. [17]	CSLO	206	OHT
Ervin et al. [18]	CSLO	24	Early POAG
Chauhan et al. [19]	CSLO	77	Early POAG
Poinoosawmy et al. [20]	SLP	110	NTG
Boehm et al. [21]	SLP	17	NTG
Mohammadi et al. [22]	SLP	160	Gl Susp
Wollstein et al. [23–25]	OCT	64	POAG

CSLO, confocal scanning laser ophthalmoscopy; SLP, scanning laser polarimetry; OCT, optical coherence tomography; OHT, ocular hypertension; POAG, primary open-angle glaucoma; NTG, normal-tension glaucoma; Gl Susp, glaucoma suspect.

photography.[14] Two technologies provide objective measures of the RNFL. With GDx with variable corneal compensation (Carl Zeiss Meditec), linearly polarized light traversing the RNFL is elliptically polarized and the amount of linear retardation of light at each corresponding retinal location is proportional to the RNFL thickness.[15] With optical coherence tomography (Status OCT, Carl Zeiss Meditec), a scanning interferometer[16] is used to obtain a cross section of the retina based on the reflectivity of the different layers of the retina. Presently, there is no accurate or reproducible way to evaluate and measure the retinal ganglion cells. There is growing evidence (Table 8-6) to suggest that these technologies can detect glaucoma progression.[17–25]

SUMMARY

Standard efficacy end points in glaucoma clinical trials include SAP and stereoscopic optic disc photography. Selective structural and functional tests have considerable advantages including high reproducibility and increased sensitivity for early glaucoma detection. They provide a potential opportunity to detect glaucoma progression earlier than standard end points, and perhaps shorten the duration of glaucoma clinical trials.

There are possible limitations to using such surrogate markers. From a regulatory perspective, it remains unclear whether these markers would be acceptable. There is currently limited clinical trial data using RNFL thickness as a surrogate end point. To differentiate biologic change from test–retest variability, confidence limits at various stages of glaucoma severity remain to be established. Finally, all technologies require further refinement and validation of software algorithms that purport to identify glaucoma.

REFERENCES

1. Keltner JL, Johnson CA, Quigg JM, et al. Confirmation of visual field abnormalities in the Ocular Hypertension Treatment Study. Ocular Hypertension Treatment Study Group. *Arch Ophthalmol* 2000;118:1187–1194.
2. Schulzer M. Errors in the diagnosis of visual field progression in normal-tension glaucoma. *Ophthalmology* 1994;101:1589–1594; discussion 1595.
3. Kass MA, Heuer DK, Higginbotham EJ, et al. The Ocular Hypertension Treatment Study: a randomized trial determines that topical ocular hypotensive medication delays or prevents the onset of primary open-angle glaucoma. *Arch Ophthalmol* 2002; 120:701–713; discussion 829–830.
4. Miglior S, Zeyen T, Pfeiffer N, et al. Results of the European Glaucoma Prevention Study. *Ophthalmology* 2005;112:366–375.
5. Heijl A, Leske MC, Bengtsson B, et al. Measuring visual field progression in the Early Manifest Glaucoma Trial. *Acta Ophthalmol Scand* 2003;81:286–293.
6. Collaborative Normal-tension Glaucoma Study Group. The effectiveness of intraocular pressure reduction in the treatment of normal-tension glaucoma. *Am J Ophthalmol* 1998; 126:498–505.
7. Collaborative Normal-tension Glaucoma Study Group. Comparison of glaucomatous progression between untreated patients with normal-tension glaucoma and patients with therapeutically reduced intraocular pressures. *Am J Ophthalmol* 1998;126:487–497.
8. Krupin T, Liebmann JM, Greenfield DS, et al. The Low-pressure Glaucoma Treatment Study (LoGTS) study design and baseline characteristics of enrolled patients. *Ophthalmology* 2005;112:376–385.
9. Medeiros FA, Sample PA, Weinreb RN. Frequency doubling technology perimetry abnormalities as predictors of glaucomatous visual field loss. *Am J Ophthalmol* 2004; 137:863–871.
10. Johnson CA, Adams AJ, Casson EJ, et al. Blue-on-yellow perimetry can predict the development of glaucomatous visual field loss. *Arch Ophthalmol* 1993;111:645–650.

11. Hood DC, Greenstein VC, Odel JG, et al. Visual field defects and multifocal visual evoked potentials: evidence of a linear relationship. *Arch Ophthalmol* 2002;120:1672–1681.

12. Porciatti V, Ventura LM. Normative data for a user-friendly paradigm for pattern electroretinogram recording. *Ophthalmology* 2004;111:161–168.

13. Zangwill LM, Weinreb RN, Beiser JA, et al. Baseline topographic optic disc measurements are associated with the development of primary open-angle glaucoma: the Confocal Scanning Laser Ophthalmoscopy Ancillary Study to the Ocular Hypertension Treatment Study. *Arch Ophthalmol* 2005;123:1188–1197.

14. Hoyt WF, Frisen L, Newman NM. Fundoscopy of nerve fiber layer defects in glaucoma. *Invest Ophthalmol* 1973;12:814–829.

15. Weinreb RN, Shakiba S, Zangwill L. Scanning laser polarimetry to measure the nerve fiber layer of normal and glaucomatous eyes. *Am J Ophthalmol* 1995;119:627–636.

16. Huang D, Swanson EA, Lin CP, et al. Optical coherence tomography. *Science* 1991;254:1178–1181.

17. Kamal DS, Garway-Heath DF, Hitchings RA, et al. Use of sequential Heidelberg retina tomograph images to identify changes at the optic disc in ocular hypertensive patients at risk of developing glaucoma. *Br J Ophthalmol* 2000;84:993–998.

18. Ervin JC, Lemij HG, Mills RP, et al. Clinician change detection viewing longitudinal stereophotographs compared to confocal scanning laser tomography in the LSU Experimental Glaucoma (LEG) Study. *Ophthalmology* 2002;109:467–481.

19. Chauhan BC, McCormick TA, Nicolela MT, et al. Optic disc and visual field changes in a prospective longitudinal study of patients with glaucoma: comparison of scanning laser tomography with conventional perimetry and optic disc photography. *Arch Ophthalmol* 2001;119:1492–1499.

20. Poinoosawmy D, Tan JC, Bunce C, et al. Longitudinal nerve fibre layer thickness change in normal-pressure glaucoma. *Graefes Arch Clin Exp Ophthalmol* 2000;238:965–969.

21. Boehm MD, Nedrud C, Greenfield DS, et al. Scanning laser polarimetry and detection of progression after optic disc hemorrhage in patients with glaucoma. *Arch Ophthalmol* 2003;121:189–194.

22. Mohammadi K, Bowd C, Weinreb RN, et al. Retinal nerve fiber layer thickness measurements with scanning laser polarimetry predict glaucomatous visual field loss. *Am J Ophthalmol* 2004;138:592–601.

23. Wollstein G, Schuman JS, Price LL, et al. Optical coherence tomography longitudinal evaluation of retinal nerve fiber layer

thickness in glaucoma. *Arch Ophthalmol* 2005; 123:464–470.

24. Wollstein G, Paunescu LA, Ko TH, et al. Ultrahigh-resolution optical coherence tomography in glaucoma. *Ophthalmology* 2005;112:229–237.

25. Wollstein G, Ishikawa H, Wang J, et al. Comparison of three optical coherence tomography scanning areas for detection of glaucomatous damage. *Am J Ophthalmol* 2005;139:39–43.

26. The AGIS Investigators. The Advanced Glaucoma Intervention Study (AGIS): 1. Study design and methods and baseline characteristics of study patients. *Control Clin Trials* 1994;15:299–325.

27. Lichter PR, Musch DC, Gillespie BW, et al. Interim clinical outcomes in the Collaborative Initial Glaucoma Treatment Study comparing initial treatment randomized to medications or surgery. *Ophthalmology* 2001;108:1943–1953.

28. Glaucoma Laser Trial Research Group. The Glaucoma Laser Trial (GLT): 6. Treatment group differences in visual field changes. *Am J Ophthalmol* 1995;120:10–22.

29. The Fluorouracil Filtering Surgery Study Group. Five-year follow-up of the Fluorouracil Filtering Surgery Study. *Am J Ophthalmol* 1996;121:349–366.

9

EVENT- AND TREND-BASED VISUAL FIELD ANALYSES IN CLINICAL TRIALS OF GLAUCOMA NEUROPROTECTION

DAVID GARWAY-HEATH, MD, FRCOphth

In glaucoma clinical trials, visual field data are collected and analyzed in various ways. This summary compares the differences between "event-based" analyses and "trend-based" analyses.[1]

An event-based method of data analysis is one in which a threshold for an event is set (Fig 9-1). When the sensitivity of a visual field test point, for instance, dips below that threshold, an event is said to have taken place. Confirmation is often required through one or more subsequent tests.

On the other hand, a trend-based method is one that looks at all the data points over time and fits a regression line (Fig. 9-2). A significant progression is usually said to have taken place if the P value is significant at a particular level and the slope attains a certain value.

Event-based change criteria have been used in all of the major clinical trials to date, including the Early Manifest Glaucoma Trial,[2] the Ocular Hypertension Treatment Study (OHTS),[3] the Collaborative Initial Glaucoma Treatment Study,[4] and the Advanced Glaucoma Intervention Study.[5] The OHTS, for example, required repeatable defects reaching a certain threshold criterion for abnormality, that is, three consecutive corrected pattern standard deviations of less than 0.05 or Glaucoma Hemifield Outside Normal Limits, with the same type, location, and index of abnormality. Similarly, the Early Manifest Glaucoma Trial required a certain, repeatable change above and beyond the baseline level of

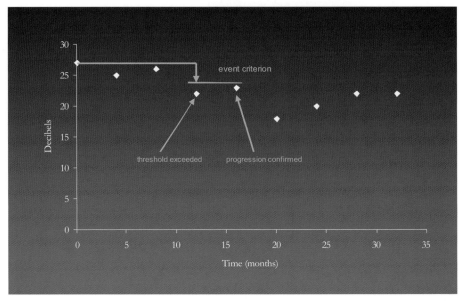

FIGURE 9-1. Event criterion: visual function in decibels, time in months, and sensitivity points over time.

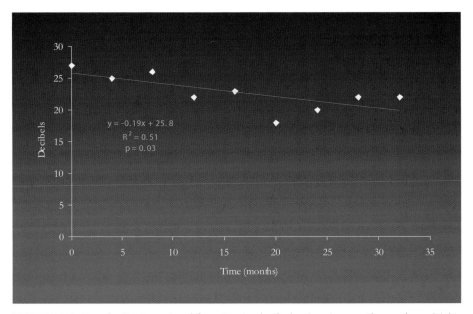

FIGURE 9-2. Trend criterion: visual function in decibels, time in months, and sensitivity points over time.

sensitivity before progression was identified. This study required at least three test points showing significant progression (on the pattern deviation Glaucoma Change Probability Maps), compared with baseline, at the same locations on three consecutive occasions.

EVENT- AND TREND-BASED METHODS: A COMPARISON

A study by Vesti et al.[6] compared the performance characteristics of seven methods for analyzing glaucomatous visual field progression. The methods included event-based methods, such as those used in the Advanced Glaucoma Intervention Study, the Collaborative Initial Glaucoma Treatment Study, and the Glaucoma Change Probability analysis, and trend-based methods that were based on pointwise linear regression analysis. The rates of progression used in the model were clinically realistic because they were taken from clinical data. For each of the methods, time to confirmed progression and sensitivity and specificity were determined under different conditions of variability. The criterion published in each study was applied to the data.

Figure 9-3 shows specificity versus the proportion of fields detected as progressing. The more specific tests tended to be less sensitive. At equivalent levels of specificity, the trend analysis tended to be more sensitive. However, the increased sensitivity was at the cost of requiring greater amounts of data. Figure 9-4 shows the time to confirmed progression versus the proportion of fields progressing. The event-based procedures tended to detect progression first, with fewer data points.

So, in comparing event-based methods with trend-based methods, the event-based methods are quicker or require fewer data points and do not assume any particular pattern of change. However, they are also wasteful of data, provide little quantification of change or rate of change information, and are inefficient. In the context of a clinical trial, the event-based methods are wasteful of data because information is gained only from the minority of patients reaching the threshold criterion for the "event." The progression status of patients not reaching the criterion is unknown, so there are fewer endpoints, which subsequently reduces the power of the study. So, more patients or a longer, more expensive study is needed to achieve more endpoints. In the OHTS, for example, only 7.6% of patients reached glaucoma endpoints, and these patients may have been progressing either quickly or slowly, depending how close to the trial endpoint they were at the start of the study. No information was obtained in the other 92.4%, who may have been progressing just as quickly or slowly, but never reached the endpoint. So information is lost, resulting in limited power to evaluate risk factors and treatment effects.

There is also little quantification in the event-based methods. The rate or magnitude of progression in individual patients is poorly summarized, again making it difficult to assess the true impact of potential risk factors and treatment effects.

Last, event-based methods are relatively inefficient. The thresholds set are usually related to population-based models of either normality or abnormality, or population-based levels of vari-

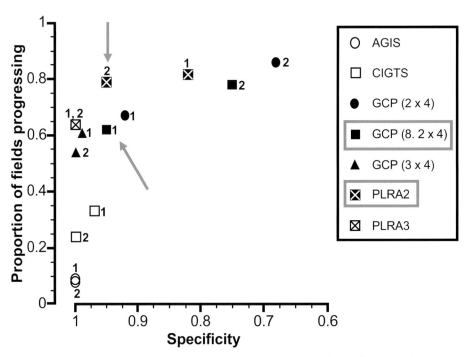

FIGURE 9-3. Proportion of progressing cases as a function of specificity for the seven methods using simulations with moderate threshold variability (1) and high threshold variability (2).

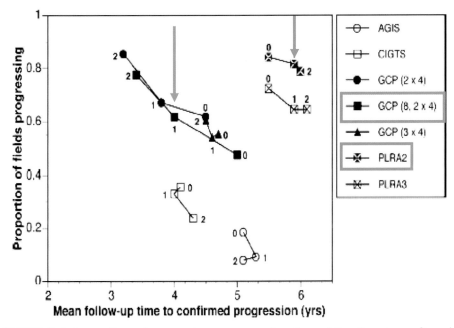

FIGURE 9-4. Proportion of progressing cases as a function of the time to confirmed progression for the seven methods using simulations with no threshold variability (*0*), moderate threshold variability (*1*), and high threshold variability (*2*).

ability, and do not use all the available data (the data between the baseline and the "event"). The problem with using population-derived limits for change is that the detection of progression may be delayed in patients with reproducible test results (it should be possible to detect smaller changes in patients with reproducible results). False-positive change may arise in patients with less reliable than average tests. Change criteria need to be revised to take into account each patient's own test reliability.

Figure 9-5 illustrates an event-based criterion requiring two confirmation fields. In this case the criterion is satisfied. If a little noise is added to the data, the patient no longer meets the conversion criterion, as illustrated in Figure 9-6. However, if the same data points are analyzed with a trend-based approach (Fig. 9-7), the slope is still significant if a little noise is added (Fig. 9-8), because all the data points are being used.

In the context of a clinical trial, however, trend-based approaches increase the study power and require fewer subjects because progression information is obtained on all subjects. These

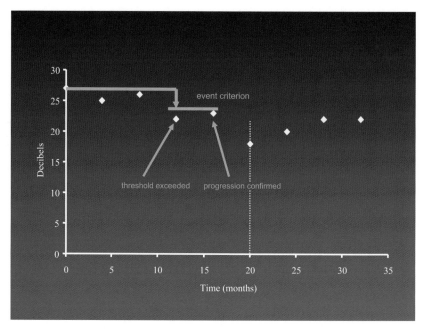

FIGURE 9-5. Visual function in decibels, time in months, and sensitivity points over time.

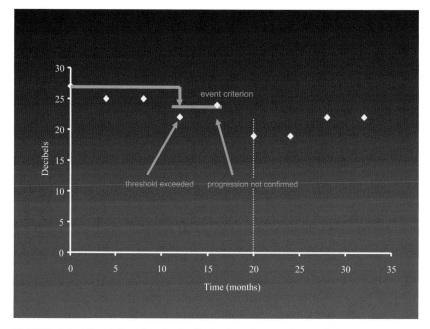

FIGURE 9-6. Visual function in decibels, time in months, and sensitivity points over time.

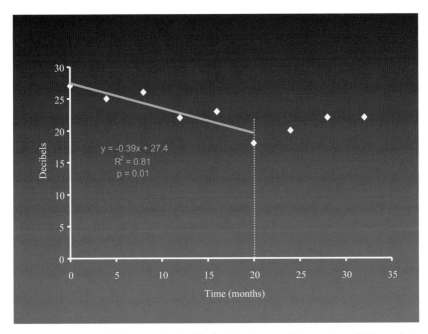

FIGURE 9-7. Visual function in decibels, time in months, and sensitivity points over time.

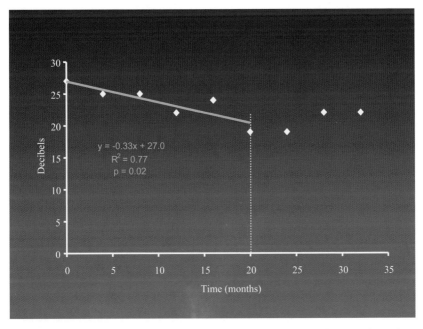

FIGURE 9-8. Visual function in decibels, time in months, and sensitivity points over time.

approaches also provide information on rate and magnitude of change. However, trend analyses either take longer or require more frequent tests over a similar duration. Trend analyses assume a consistent linear progression, although stepwise progression may be detected.

RATE-BASED METHODS

Rate-based methods of measuring progression allow for the assessment of mean deviation (MD) of the visual field over time, mean sensitivity over time, or pointwise sensitivity over time. Studies looking at MD over time have largely reported poor sensitivity.[7–9] However, these are clinical studies and, by their nature, have no external "gold standard" by which to define stability or progression of the visual field.

Two studies that examined visual field sectors over time have reported better sensitivity.[7,9] The first, by Smith et al.,[7] included 191 patients with glaucomatous visual field loss and a minimum of seven threshold field tests over at least 4.5 years. Higher hit rates were found with clusterwise and pointwise forms of analysis over the analysis of summary parameters (12.6% significant MD slope, 14.1% significant corrected pattern standard deviation slope, 18.3% significant Glaucoma Hemifield Test cluster slope, 18.8% significant single location slope).

Another study, by Nouri-Mahdavi et al.,[9] consisted of clinical evaluations of 83 patients with open-angle glaucoma and five or more eligible fields. The data from this study indicated that visual field summary variables were not particularly useful. Pointwise and clusterwise methods were better and comparable.

Modeling techniques have been used to evaluate pointwise progression detection with the "three-omitting" criterion, which uses two confirmation fields in a novel way.[10] Test point sensitivity is analyzed over time, and the progression criterion is satisfied when a significant slope is identified in all of the following: (1) at a test point in visual field "n" in a time series, (2) at the same test point when visual field "n" is omitted and visual field n+1 is included, and (3) at the same test point when visual fields "n" and "n+1" are omitted and visual field n+2 is included. This approach improved specificity when compared with the standard criteria, and maintained high sensitivity for detecting progression.

When pointwise linear regression is applied in practice, PROGRESSOR software developed by Viswanathan et al.[11] can be used. Progression indices include the number of progressing points, mean slope for the whole field (dB/year), and mean slope for progressing points (dB/year). This technique was applied by Bhandari et al.[12] in a study of 17 patients with normal tension glaucoma who were found to be progressing and subsequently underwent surgery. This method demonstrated a significant reduction in the rate of progression after, compared with before, surgery.

A potential experimental design is illustrated in Figure 9-9. Patients who are progressing rapidly are identified ("observation phase") and randomized to the treatment options. The progression slopes before and after the intervention, or between the two interventions, may be compared. Progression slopes may be analyzed on a pointwise, clusterwise, or whole-field (mean sensitivity) basis. In the observation phase, using cluster criteria, progression was defined as at least one cluster progressing at P less than .01, or two ad-

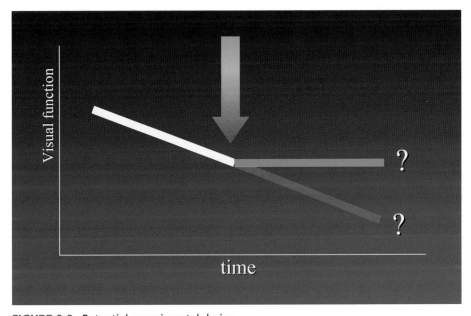

FIGURE 9-9. Potential experimental design.

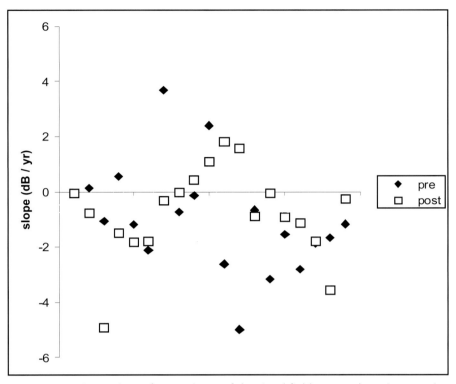

FIGURE 9-10. Comparison of mean slopes of the visual field, pre- and postintervention.

jacent clusters progressing at between $P = .01$ and $P = .05$ during the 18-month observation phase. Decreased or stopped progression was defined as the slope of previously progressing cluster(s) decreased by at least 50%, and no further clusters showing progression. By using the PROGRESSOR software, the mean slope of the visual field may be analyzed and a comparison may be made between the pre- and postintervention slopes (Fig. 9-10).

A key feature of the rate-based method is that the rate of progression, which may be a trial primary outcome, is measured in all subjects, thus improving the power of the study while requiring fewer patients in the study. The progression rate can be measured in a shorter period if the rate of progression is faster. So, inclusion of patients who are at higher risk of progression, that is, those progressing faster at baseline (during the observation period), in a rate-based study design may allow the detection of treatment effects in a relatively short period with relatively few subjects.

SUMMARY

Rate-based methods seem to be highly suitable for visual field outcome measurement in randomized controlled trials. Further work is needed to elucidate the best way to combine summary, clusterwise, or pointwise methods and to determine the optimal pattern and frequency of acquiring the data from patients, individualized on the basis of the noise characteristics of each patient.

REFERENCES

1. Artes PH, Chauhan BC. Longitudinal changes in the visual field and optic disc in glaucoma. *Prog Retin Eye Res* 2005;24:333–354.
2. Heijl A, Leske MC, Bengtsson B, et al. Measuring visual field progression in the Early Manifest Glaucoma Trial. *Acta Ophthalmol Scand* 2003;81:286–293.
3. Kass MA, Heuer DK, Higginbotham EJ, et al. The Ocular Hypertension Treatment Study: a randomized trial determines that topical ocular hypotensive medication delays or prevents the onset of primary open-angle glaucoma. *Arch Ophthalmol* 2002;120:701–713; discussion 829–830.
4. Lichter PR, Musch DC, Gillespie BW, et al. Interim clinical outcomes in the Collaborative Initial Glaucoma Treatment Study comparing initial treatment randomized to medications or surgery. *Ophthalmology* 2001;108:1943–1953.
5. The AGIS Investigators. The Advanced Glaucoma Intervention Study (AGIS): 1. Study design and methods and baseline characteristics of study patients. *Control Clin Trials* 1994;15:299–325.
6. Vesti E, Johnson CA, Chauhan BC. Comparison of different methods for detecting glaucomatous visual field progression. *Invest Ophthalmol Vis Sci* 2003;44:3873–3879.
7. Smith SD, Katz J, Quigley HA. Analysis of progressive change in automated visual fields in glaucoma. *Invest Ophthalmol Vis Sci* 1996;37:1419–1428.
8. Wild JM, Hutchings N, Hussey MK, et al. Pointwise univariate linear regression of perimetric sensitivity against follow-up time

in glaucoma. *Ophthalmology* 1997;104:808–815.

9. Nouri-Mahdavi K, Brigatti L, Weitzman M, et al. Comparison of methods to detect visual field progression in glaucoma. *Ophthalmology* 1997;104:1228–1236.

10. Gardiner SK, Crabb DP. Examination of different pointwise linear regression methods for determining visual field progression. *Invest Ophthalmol Vis Sci* 2002;43:1400–1407.

11. Viswanathan AC, Fitzke FW, Hitchings RA. Early detection of visual field progression in glaucoma: a comparison of PROGRESSOR and STATPAC 2. *Br J Ophthalmol* 1997;81:1037–1042.

12. Bhandari A, Crabb DP, Poinoosawmy D, et al. Effect of surgery on visual field progression in normal-tension glaucoma. *Ophthalmology* 1997;104:1131–1137.

10

THE LOW-PRESSURE GLAUCOMA TREATMENT STUDY: PROTOCOL AND BASELINE CHARACTERISTICS

THEODORE KRUPIN, MD, AND JEFFREY M. LIEBMANN, MD

The definition of glaucoma has gone through a number of changes in the last few years. In the last edition of *The Glaucomas*,[1] the condition was described as "an optic neuropathy characterized by a specific pattern of optic nerve head and visual field damage, which represents a final common pathway resulting from a number of different conditions that can affect the eye . . . most (but not all) of which cause elevated intraocular pressure." Although elevated intraocular pressure (IOP) is recognized as the most important risk factor for the development or progression of glaucomatous damage, it is still considered as only a risk factor and not the disease per se. The American Academy of Ophthalmology's Preferred Practice Patterns defines glaucoma as a "multifactorial optic neuropathy characterized by acquired loss of retinal ganglion cells and optic nerve atrophy." In this document, there is a conspicuous absence of any reference to IOP, until much further along in the text.

Obviously, low- and high-pressure open-angle glaucoma are a continuum and cannot be separated by a single IOP level. At present, we are unable to determine an individual's optic nerve susceptibility to any given level of IOP. Patients show marked variation in the degree of harm caused by a given IOP, as well as a wide variation in the level of IOP tolerated without harm. In low-pressure glaucoma (LPG), pressure-independent mechanisms (e.g., genetic, vascular, biologic, or structural defects of the retinal ganglion cell or optic nerve) may be the main, if not the sole, causes of the optic neuropathy. Thus, the study of patients with LPG provides a means to investigate some of these mechanisms in glaucomatous optic neuropathy.

The term "low-pressure glaucoma" does exist and has been given many different names, including "pseudoglaucoma,"[2] "low-tension glaucoma," glaucoma with normal pressure,"[3] and "normal tension glaucoma." My preference is "low-pressure glaucoma," rather than "normal tension glaucoma." The term "normal"—which means statistically normal, but not pathologically normal—is difficult to use when discussing the condition with a patient worried about blindness. The only "tension" involved is that experienced by the patient and the ophthalmologist in facing this condition.

LOW-PRESSURE GLAUCOMA TREATMENT STUDY

The Low-pressure Glaucoma Treatment Study (LoGTS) is a double-masked, multicenter, randomized clinical trial designed to compare the course of patients with LPG randomized to IOP reduction with topical twice-daily brimonidine tartrate 0.2% versus twice-daily timolol maleate 0.5%. The study was supported by an unrestricted grant from Allergan, Inc. (Irvine, CA). Study investigators are listed in Table 10-1. The remainder of this discussion will summarize the study protocol and baseline characteristics of study participants.[4]

Subjects included 190 men and women, aged 30 years or more, with previously diagnosed LPG in at least one eye, and untreated IOP of 21 mm Hg or less on an 8-hour IOP pressure curve (8:00 A.M., 10:00 A.M., noon, and 4:00 P.M.) on day zero. The diagnosis of LPG required open iridocorneal angles by gonioscopy and glaucomatous visual field defects in at least one eye on Humphrey 24-2 full-threshold standard automatic perimetry. At least two visual field examinations with acceptable reliability standards were required within the prior 6 months. Vision of at least 20/40 was also required. Pseudophakia was allowed if surgery was performed more than 1 year earlier.

The pertinent exclusion criteria included a history of treated or untreated IOP greater than 21 mm Hg, untreated IOP greater

TABLE 10-1. LOW-PRESSURE GLAUCOMA STUDY GROUP INVESTIGATORS

University Eye Specialists, Chicago, Illinois
Theodore Krupin, MD, Lisa F. Rosenberg, MD, Jon M. Ruderman, MD, John W. Yang, MD, and Lucilla Gonzalez (LoGTS coordinator)

New York Eye & Ear Infirmary, New York, New York
Celso Tello, MD, Jeffrey M. Liebmann, MD, Robert Ritch, MD

Wills Eye Hospital, Philadelphia, Pennsylvania
Jonathan S. Myers, MD, L. Jay Katz, MD, George L. Spaeth, MD, Douglas J. Rhee, MD, Richard P. Wilson, MD, and Marlene R. Moster, MD

Indiana University, Indianapolis, Indiana
Louis B. Cantor, MD

Cullen Eye Institute, Baylor College, Houston, Texas
Ronald L. Gross, MD

Rapid City, South Dakota
Monte S. Dirks, MD

Brooke Army Medical Center, San Antonio, Texas
Steven R. Grimes, MD

Bascom Palmer Eye Institute, University of Miami School of Medicine, Palm Beach Gardens, Florida
David S. Greenfield, MD, and Harmohina Bagga, MD

University of Florida, Gainesville, Florida
Mark B. Sherwood, MD

University of Chicago, Chicago, Illinois
Marianne E. Feitl, MD

Little Rock Eye Clinic, Little Rock, Arkansas
J. Charles Henry, MD

Wheaton Eye Clinic, Wheaton, Illinois
David K. Gieser, MD

Scheie Eye Institute, University of Pennsylvania, Philadelphia, Pennsylvania
Jody R. Piltz-Seymour, MD

than 21 mm Hg in an 8-hour IOP curve, or a greater than 4 mm Hg IOP difference between the eyes. Patients with advanced glaucoma (mean deviation, 15 decibels) were also excluded, as well as those with evidence of exfoliation, pigment dispersion, or prior filtration surgery.

The primary end point was visual field. Patients were examined at 1 and 4 months after initiation of treatment randomization and every 4 months (±2 weeks) thereafter. Baseline visual field was defined as the average of two prerandomization examinations. Optic disks were evaluated by physician assessment every 4 months and by photographs at baseline and every year thereafter. Photographs were evaluated at the Optic Disc Reading Center. Central corneal thickness (CCT) was also measured.

Age

The average patient age was 64.9 ± 10.7 years (mean ± standard deviation). Twenty-two patients (11.6%) were aged less than 50 years (Fig. 10-1). The Beaver Dam Eye Study[5] showed earlier that the prevalence of LPG increased with age, from 0.2% in the group aged 43 to 54 years to 1.6% in the group aged more than 75 years, with 63.6% of the patients aged more than 64 years. In the LoGTS, only 54.2% of patients were aged more than 64 years, a smaller percentage than in the Beaver Dam Study. This may relate to improved clin-

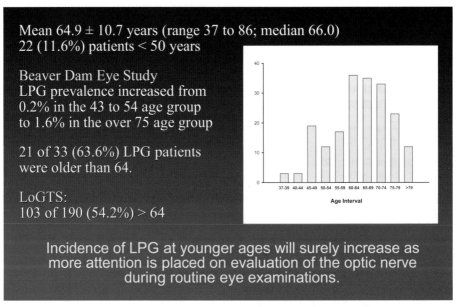

Mean 64.9 ± 10.7 years (range 37 to 86; median 66.0)
22 (11.6%) patients < 50 years

Beaver Dam Eye Study
LPG prevalence increased from
0.2% in the 43 to 54 age group
to 1.6% in the over 75 age group

21 of 33 (63.6%) LPG patients
were older than 64.

LoGTS:
103 of 190 (54.2%) > 64

Incidence of LPG at younger ages will surely increase as
more attention is placed on evaluation of the optic nerve
during routine eye examinations.

FIGURE 10-1. Patient demographics: age distribution of LoPGT study patients. (Source: Krupin T, Liebmann JM, Greenfield DS, et al. The Low-pressure Glaucoma Treatment Study (LoGTS) study design and baseline characteristics of enrolled patients. *Ophthalmology* 2005;112:376–385.)

ical evaluation of the optic nerve. The incidence of LPG at younger ages will surely increase as more attention is placed on evaluation of the optic nerve during routine eye examinations.

Sex

There were more women (n = 113; 59.5%) than men (n = 77; 40.5%; *P* = .0003) with LPG. Earlier reports on gender distribution of LPG have reported greater frequency in women,[6,7] greater frequency in men,[8] or an equal distribution between the sexes.[5]

Family History

Earlier findings also reported that 40% of patients with LPG had a history of chronic open-angle glaucoma (COAG).[9] In the LoGTS, 30% of the patients had a family history of COAG, and a few (4%) had a family history of LPG.

A history of migraine headaches was reported in nine participants (4.7%), a finding similar to earlier findings in the Beaver Dam Study[5] and a study by Lewis et al.[10] In 1985, Phelps and Corbett[11] reported a 37% incidence of migraine in patients with LPG, higher than in healthy subjects or patients with COAG by approximately 22%.

Although previous reports in the literature cited a high occurrence of functional peripheral vasospasm (up to ~65%),[12,13] only 16 LoGTS participants (8.4%) reported a history compatible with Raynaud's phenomenon.

Visual Field Loss

Visual field defects in both eyes were present in 137 patients (72.1%); unilateral defects were present in 53 patients (27.9%) at baseline, with the left eye more commonly involved (56.6%). This is similar to the 25% occurrence of unilateral field loss (64% in the left eye) in LPG reported by Poinoosawmy et al.[14]

The patients with unilateral field loss were younger than the patients with bilateral field loss, with the proportion of unilateral cases decreasing with increasing age (Fig. 10-2). The younger age of these patients may relate to the earlier detection of optic nerve damage in those with a normal IOP.

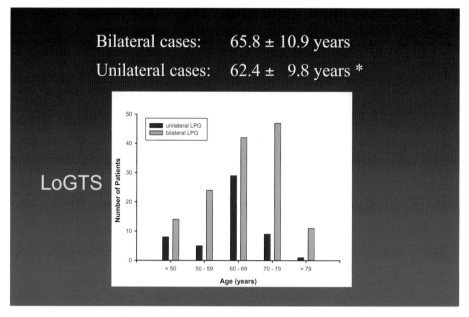

FIGURE 10-2. Ocular findings: field loss minus age. Age distribution of bilateral versus unilateral field loss in LoPGT study patients. Percentage of participants aged more than 64 years: total, 56.3% (107/190); bilateral visual field loss, 59.8% (82/137); unilateral visual field loss 47.2% (25/53). Unilateral LPG, patients with unilateral field loss; bilateral LPG, patients with bilateral field loss. (Source: Krupin T, Liebmann JM, Greenfield DS, et al. The Low-pressure Glaucoma Treatment Study (LoGTS) study design and baseline characteristics of enrolled patients. *Ophthalmology* 2005;112:376–385.)

Cupping

As expected, cup-to-disc ratios in the participants with unilateral field loss were higher ($P < .0001$) in the eyes with field loss than in the fellow eyes without visual field damage.

Intraocular Pressure

The mean of the four baseline pressure readings of nontreated IOP was equal in both eyes (Table 10-2). There was no difference between eyes in the mean nontreated 8-hour IOP curve of the 137 patients with bilateral field loss. There were 18 patients with bilateral field loss who had some asymmetry in pressure. Nontreated day 0 IOP curve was similar between the eyes of the 53 subjects with unilateral field loss. Most eyes were equal in IOP by 1 mm

TABLE 10-2. BASELINE 8-HOUR INTRAOCULAR PRESSURE MEASUREMENTS

Time	Right Eyes* (mm Hg)	Left Eyes* (mm Hg)
8:00 AM	15.9 ± 2.8 (10.0–21.0; 15.5, 16.3)	16.0 ± 2.7 (8.0–20.5; 15.7, 16.3)
10:00 AM	15.5 ± 2.7 (9.5–20.5; 15.1, 15.9)	15.6 ± 2.8 (7.5–21.0; 15.2, 16)
12:00 PM	15.5 ± 2.6 (8.0–20.5; 15.1, 15.9)	15.6 ± 2.6 (8.0–20.5; 15.2, 15.9)
4:00 PM	14.9 ± 2.8 (8.5–20.0; 14.9, 15.7)	15.4 ± 2.8 (8.0–20.5; 15.0, 15.8)

*Mean ± standard deviation (range; 95% confidence intervals).
(Source: Krupin T, Liebmann JM, Greenfield DS, et al. The Low-pressure Glaucoma Treatment Study (LoGTS) study design and baseline characteristics of enrolled patients. *Ophthalmology* 2005;112:376–385.)

Hg, although there were 12 subjects who had higher pressure in the field loss eye and 8 subjects who had lower pressure in the field loss eye.

Corneal Thickness

CCT was measured in 168 of 171 phakic patients. Mean CCT ranged from 435 to 655 μm. CCT was less than 500 μm in 15 patients (30 eyes; 8.9%) and more than 600 μm in 11 patients (22 eyes; 7.1%). There was no statistically significant difference in CCT between the patients with bilateral field loss and the patients with unilateral field loss. The impact of corneal thickness obviously is that thin CCTs can underestimate the true IOP and can classify a patient inaccurately as having LPG (IOP <22 mm Hg in our study). Shah et al.[15] previously reported low mean CCTs in 52 of 514 patients with LPG. The LoGTS does not confirm an excess of thin corneas in patients with LPG.

SUMMARY

The baseline characteristics of this large group of patients with LPG enrolled in the prospective LoGTS clinical trial provide useful information on IOP, visual field loss, and optic nerve hemorrhages. These data can help to formulate better treatment paradigms for patients with open angle glaucoma with relatively low IOPs.

REFERENCES

1. Ritch R, Shields MB, Krupin T, eds. *The glaucomas.* St. Louis, MO: CV Mosby Co; 1996.
2. Sjogren H. The nature of pseudoglaucoma. *N Z Med J* 1952;51:(Suppl)14–21.
3. Drance SM. Low-tension glaucoma. Enigma and opportunity. *Arch Ophthalmol* 1985; 103:1131–1133.
4. Krupin T, Liebmann JM, Greenfield DS, et al. The Low-pressure Glaucoma Treatment Study (LoGTS) study design and baseline characteristics of enrolled patients. *Ophthalmology* 2005;112:376–385.
5. Klein BE, Klein R, Sponsel WE, et al. Prevalence of glaucoma. The Beaver Dam Eye Study. *Ophthalmology* 1992;99:1499–1504.
6. Chumbley LC, Brubaker RF. Low-tension glaucoma. *Am J Ophthalmol* 1976;81: 761–767.
7. Goldberg I, Hollows FC, Kass MA, et al. Systemic factors in patients with low-tension glaucoma. *Br J Ophthalmol* 1981;65:56–62.
8. Drance SM, Sweeney VP, Morgan RW, et al. Studies of factors involved in the production of low tension glaucoma. *Arch Ophthalmol* 1973;89:457–465.
9. Geijssen HC. *Studies on normal-pressure glaucoma.* The Netherlands: Kugler; 1991.
10. Lewis RA, Hayreh SS, Phelps CD. Optic disk and visual field correlations in primary open-angle and low-tension glaucoma. *Am J Ophthalmol* 1983;96:148–152.
11. Phelps CD, Corbett JJ. Migraine and low-tension glaucoma. A case-control study. *Invest Ophthalmol Vis Sci* 1985;26:1105–1108.
12. Drance SM, Morgan RW, Sweeney VP. Shock-induced optic neuropathy: a cause of nonprogressive glaucoma. *N Engl J Med* 1973;288:392–395.
13. Gasser P, Flammer J. Influence of vasospasm on visual function. *Doc Ophthalmol* 1987;66:3–18.
14. Poinoosawmy D, Fontana L, Wu JX, et al. Frequency of asymmetric visual field defects in normal-tension and high-tension glaucoma. *Ophthalmology* 1998;105:988–991.
15. Shah S, Chatterjee A, Mathai M, et al. Relationship between corneal thickness and measured intraocular pressure in a general ophthalmology clinic. *Ophthalmology* 1999; 106:2154–2160.

Index

GLAUCOMA NEUROPROTECTION

POST TEST

To earn CME credit, a participant must read the monograph, comprehend the content, and complete the CME quiz and evaluation assessment survey on form printed at the end of the book, answering at least 70% of the CME quiz questions correctly. Participants must make a photocopy of the completed answer form for their own files and <u>send their original answer form</u> to Wolters Kluwer Health, Office of Continuing Education, 770 Township Line Road, Suite 300, Yardley, PA 19067. Only the first entry will be considered for credit and must be received by WKH by 2/28/2008. **Acknowledgment will be sent to participants within 6 to 8 weeks of participation. AMA/PRA Category 1 credit is available** <u>**only**</u> **to U.S.-licensed physicians (MDs or DOs). All other healthcare professionals who return the quiz and achieve a passing score will receive a certificate of completion for successful participation.**

Wolters Kluwer Health is accredited by the Accreditation Council for Continuing Medical Education to provide continuing medical education for physicians.

Wolters Kluwer Health designates this educational activity for up to 5 category 1 credits toward the AMA Physician's Recognition Award. Each physician should claim only those credits that he/she actually spent in the activity.

1. Glaucoma is unlikely to progress significantly if a low level of intraocular pressure (IOP) can be maintained.
   a. True
   b. False

2. In general, most optic neuropathies involve:
   a. The axon but not the cell body
   b. Both the axon and the cell body
   c. The cell body but not the axon

3. Which of the following neuroprotective agents have been shown to block excessive activation of the NMDA receptor while leaving normal function relatively intact?
   a. memantine
   b. MK-801
   c. ketamine
   d. all of the above
   e. none of the above

4. Under physiological conditions, memantine has a very high affinity for the NMDA receptor.
   a. True
   b. False

5. The amantadine derivative memantine blocks the NMDA receptor-operated channels very effectively:
   a. Only when the channels are excessively open (i.e., when there is more glutamate in the channel)
   b. Only under normal physiological conditions
   c. Under both pathological and normal conditions
   d. Only when levels of receptor activity are very low

6. Memantine is effective in blocking what percentage of normal neurotransmission?
   a. 0%
   b. 5%
   c. 30%
   d. 50%
   e. 90% or more

7. In placebo-controlled clinical trials of Alzheimer's disease patients, the use of memantine (either alone or with a cholinesterase inhibitor) resulted in significantly better outcomes in measures of:
   a. Cognition, but not function
   b. Function, but not cognition
   c. Both cognition and function
   d. Neither cognition nor function

8. Clinical researchers have attempted to assess neuroprotective effects of drug treatment by measuring the drug's effect on cerebral glucose metabolism.
   a. True
   b. False

9. In the retina, glutamate is released by:
   a. Ganglion cells
   b. Photoreceptors
   c. Bipolar cells
   d. All of the above
   e. None of the above

10. In preclinical trials, administration of memantine was associated with significant consistent reductions in intraocular pressure.
    a. True
    b. False

11. The primary injury in glaucoma is at the level of the:
    a. Visual cortex
    b. Lateral geniculate nucleus
    c. Retinal ganglion cells
    d. None of the above

12. Most optic nerve fibers that arise from retinal ganglion cells terminate in the lateral geniculate nucleus.
    a. True
    b. False

13. Neural degeneration may result from:
    a. Nerve growth factor deprivation
    b. Autoimmune reactions
    c. Oxidative damage
    d. Glutamate excitotoxicity
    e. All of the above

14. Memantine is currently FDA-approved for the treatment of:
    a. Parkinson's disease
    b. Vascular dementia
    c. Alzheimer's disease
    d. Open-angle glaucoma
    e. All of the above

15. In general, activation of the alpha-2 adrenergic receptors tends to "turn up" the activity of the nervous system.
    a. True
    b. False

16. Brimonidine is a selective alpha-2 agonist that is currently used to lower IOP in glaucoma patients.
    a. True
    b. False

17. In preclinical neuroprotection studies, which of the following has been used as a marker of retinotectal projection and anterograde axonal transport?
    a. Brimonidine
    b. Cholera toxin subunit-B
    c. Timolol
    d. Glial fibrillary acidic protein

18. In preclinical trials, topical administration of brimonidine provided neuroprotection against retinal ischemia, but only when administered before the injury.
    a. True
    b. False

19. In preclinical trials, the alpha-2 agonist brimonidine, prevented or diminished ischemia-induced alterations of the inner and outer retinal ganglion cell layers, as well as the main retinofugal projection.
    a. True
    b. False

20. Generally, only one efficacy endpoint is necessary to establish visual field progression, as long as the endpoint has been well-validated.
    a. True
    b. False

21. The assessment of visual function in glaucoma that uses a blue target presented on a yellow background and measures koniocellular retinal ganglion cell function is known as:
    a. SAP (standard automated perimetry)
    b. SWAP (short-wavelength automated perimetry)

c. FDT (frequency doubling technology)
d. Multifocal visual evoked potential testing
e. None of the above

22. The Heidelberg Retinal Tomograph, a confocal scanning laser ophthalmoscope, has been shown to predict conversion to primary open-angle glaucoma with a power of about:
    a. <10%
    b. 25%
    c. 40%
    d. 75%
    e. >90%

23. In general, event-based methods of visual field data analysis, when compared with trend-based methods:
    a. Are slower
    b. Require more data points
    c. Provide little quantification of change
    e. All of the above

24. Rate-based methods of measuring visual field progression allow for the assessment of:
    a. Mean deviation (MD) over time
    b. Mean sensitivity over time
    c. Pointwise sensitivity over time
    d. All of the above
    e. None of the above

25. Patients with glaucoma generally show a marked consistency in the level of intraocular pressure (IOP) tolerated without harm.
    a. True
    b. False

CME EXAMINATION
QUIZ ANSWER SHEET

FIRST NAME _____ LAST NAME _____

HIGHEST EDUCATIONAL DEGREE _____

ADDRESS _____

_____

CITY/STATE/ZIP _____

PHONE NUMBER _____

Please mark box with check or X. Do not fill in boxes completely:

	A	B	C	D	E
1.	☐	☐	☐	☐	☐
2.	☐	☐	☐	☐	☐
3.	☐	☐	☐	☐	☐
4.	☐	☐	☐	☐	☐
5.	☐	☐	☐	☐	☐
6.	☐	☐	☐	☐	☐
7.	☐	☐	☐	☐	☐
8.	☐	☐	☐	☐	☐
9.	☐	☐	☐	☐	☐
10.	☐	☐	☐	☐	☐
11.	☐	☐	☐	☐	☐
12.	☐	☐	☐	☐	☐
13.	☐	☐	☐	☐	☐
14.	☐	☐	☐	☐	☐
15.	☐	☐	☐	☐	☐
16.	☐	☐	☐	☐	☐

	A	B	C	D	E
17.	☐	☐	☐	☐	☐
18.	☐	☐	☐	☐	☐
19.	☐	☐	☐	☐	☐
20.	☐	☐	☐	☐	☐
21.	☐	☐	☐	☐	☐
22.	☐	☐	☐	☐	☐
23.	☐	☐	☐	☐	☐
24.	☐	☐	☐	☐	☐
25.	☐	☐	☐	☐	☐

EVALUATION ASSESSMENT FORM

Your evaluation of this CME activity will help guide future planning. Please respond to the following questions:

1. Did the content of this activity meet the stated learning objectives?
   [ ] Yes   [ ] No

2. As a result of meeting the learning objectives of the educational activity, will you be changing your practice behavior in a manner that improves your patient care? If yes, please explain.
   [ ] Yes   [ ] No

   _____

   _____

   _____

   _____

   _____

3. On a scale of 1 to 5, with 5 being the highest, how do you rank the overall quality of this educational activity?
   [ ] 5   [ ] 4   [ ] 3   [ ] 2   [ ] 1

4. Did you perceive any evidence of bias for or against any commercial products in this activity? If yes, please explain.
   [ ] Yes   [ ] No

   _____

   _____

   _____

   _____

   _____

5. Please state 1 or 2 topics that you would like to see addressed in future educational activities.

   _____

   _____

   _____

   _____

   _____

6. How long did it take you to complete this activity? _____ hours